Low Fat Cooking

Lose Fat with Clean Eating and the Belly Fat Diet

Margarete Aguilera and Tabitha Stich

Copyright © 2013 Margarete Aguilera and Tabitha Stich
All rights reserved.

Table of Contents

INTRODUCTION 1

SECTION 1: CLEAN EATING 6

CHAPTER 1: THE CLEAN DIET 10

CHAPTER 3: ALTERNATIVE FOOD TYPES 17

CHAPTER 4: TIPS FOR EATING CLEAN AND HEALTHY 21

CHAPTER 5: 5-DAY SAMPLE PLANNER FOR DAY TO DAY MEALS 23

CHAPTER 6: BREAKFAST RECIPES 27
- Breakfast Fiesta..27
- Rise and Shine Banana Bread 29
- Sweet and Zesty Pancake Apple Rings 31
- Healthy Granola Breakfast Cereal.....................................33
- Springtime Baked Omelet..35

CHAPTER 7: QUICK AND EASY LUNCHES.................. 37
- Reuben Supreme Sandwich..37
- Creamy Albacore Pita 38
- Touch of Italy Cheese Quesadillas....................................40
- Greens and Berries Super Salad 42
- Marinated Salmon with Cucumber Salsa 44

CHAPTER 8: MAIN MEAL RECIPES 46
- Beef Asparagus Stir-Fry..46
- Home Made Beef Tacos with Salsa 48

Crispy Fish Fillets with Lemon Dip 51
Thick and Chunky Oven Chili 53
Savory Scallops with Zesty Spinach 55
No Problem Grilled Jerk Chicken 57

CHAPTER 9: SIDE DISHES 59
Cauliflower Fanfare 59
Quinoa Corn Salad 61
Stuffed Zucchini Boats 63
Sassy Apricots and Sweet Potatoes 65
Spring Pea-Cheddar Salad 67
Green Bean Casserole Supreme 69

CHAPTER 10: DESSERTS 71
Original Angel Food Cake 71
Raspberry-Peach Crumble 73
Classy Carrot Cake 75
Lemon Bundt Cake with Poppy Seeds 77
Peanut Butter Cookies-Hold the Flour 80
Perfect Strawberry Parfait 82

CHAPTER 11: SNACKS 84
Caribbean Fruitsicles 84
Snackin' Cranberry Granola 86
Vanilla Lovers Granola 88
Bugs on a Log 90
Apple-Cinnamon Chips 91
Fruit-Nutty Trail Mix 93

CHAPTER 12: BEVERAGES 95
Green Tea/Mango Surprise 95
Homemade Honey Lemonade 96
Peachy Spritzer 98
Famous Fruity Smoothie 99
Chocolate Covered Banana Milkshake 100
Honeydew Delight 101
Caribbean Cooler 102

CLEAN EATING CONCLUSION 103

SECTION 2: BELLY FAT DIET 105

CHAPTER 1: WHAT IS THE BELLY FAT DIET? 107

The Secret Behind the Diet 107

How the Diet Works 108

CHAPTER 2: BENEFITS OF THE BELLY FAT DIET 110

CHAPTER 3: ESSENTIAL TIPS FOR SUCCESS ON THE BELLY MELT DIET 113

Helpful Diet Tips to Follow 113

Top Belly Fat Burning Foods 115

CHAPTER 4: BELLY MELTING BREAKFAST RECIPES 118

Banana Walnut Breakfast Muffin Recipe 119
Tomato Pesto Eggs Florentine Breakfast Recipe 121
Pumpkin Pie Flavored Oatmeal Breakfast Recipe 123
Delicious French Toast with Chocolate Breakfast Recipe 125
Belly Melt Huevos Racheros Breakfast Recipe 127
Belly Filling Parfait with Granola Breakfast Recipe 129
Decadent Walnut Banana Pancakes Breakfast Recipe 130
Pecan and Cranberry Scones Breakfast Recipe 132
Nut and Fruit Oatmeal Breakfast Recipe 134

CHAPTER 5: GREAT LUNCH RECIPES TO HELP YOU LOSE BELLY FAT 136

Easy Turkey Pita with Side Salad Lunch Recipe 137
Shrimp, Barley and Baby Green Salad Lunch Recipe 139
Rainbow Veggie, Soba Noodle and Chicken Salad Lunch Recipe 141
Mediterranean Style Wraps Lunch Recipe 143

Low Sugar Strawberry and Peanut Butter Wraps Lunch Recipe 145
Easy Whole Wheat Muffin Pizzas Lunch Recipe 147
Walnut and Radish Spinach Salad Lunch Recipe 149

CHAPTER 6: FLAT BELLY DIET DINNER RECIPES 151
Smoked Salmon Frittata Dinner Recipe 152
Chicken Breast with Almond Crust Dinner Recipe 154
Easy Belly Busting Slow Cooker Chili Dinner Recipe................................ 156
Snow Peas and Steamed Gingered Salmon Dinner Recipe 158
Chicken Roulade Stuffed with Spinach Dinner Recipe 160
Easy Whole Wheat Veggie Pizza Recipe 163
Roasted Pepper and Portobello Mushroom Burgers Recipe 165
Pepper Steak Tacos Dinner Recipe 167
Belly Flattening Broccoli Rabe Sausage Penne Recipe 170

CHAPTER 7: BELLY FLATTENING DRINK, SNACK AND DESSERT RECIPES 173
Ricotta and Citrus Cannoli Dessert Recipe.. 173
Tasty Strawberry Tropical Fruit Smoothie Recipe 175
Delicious Apple Yogurt Dessert Recipe 177
Mocha Protein Health Snack Bites Recipe 179
Delicious Peanut Butter Balls Recipe 181

CHAPTER 8: YOUR 7 DAY BELLY FAT DIET MEAL PLAN 183

Introduction

You bought this book because you wish to go on a low fat diet. There are two diets represented here that offer recipes that are naturally low in fat, the clean eating diet, and the belly fat diet. Each of these diets offers recipes that call for healthy nutritious foods like fresh fruits and vegetables, whole grains, lean meats and savory herbs. By going on a diet that is low in fat, you can safely lose weight while toning the body to become healthier.

To make the dieting successful you need to determine right now that this will be a lifestyle change. If you just diet long enough to lose the weight then go back to your same old bad eating habits, the weight and fat will pile right back on your body. But if you lose the weight, then make the way you eat a permanent change you will be able to maintain the weight loss better. Other things you can do will prepare for the diet and make the diet a success.

The first things you will want to do before starting a successful diet is to break your bad habits. Bad habits are health suckers, they make the immune system weak and cause you to be sick more. If you can break these before you diet, you will not have to focus on withdrawal symptoms, because you will already be over it. Bad habits that are detrimental to your health are smoking, excessive alcohol drinking, addiction to junk food, recreational drugs, and caffeine. All of these rob your health. Take the time to wean from each one so you can put all your focus on your diet. Sometimes it can take a while to turn your lifestyle around for the better.

While you are breaking the bad habits, go ahead and eat the foods on these diets, but if you are breaking bad habits work on those first. Start breaking the worse of the bad habits first. If you are addicted to recreational drugs, this is the right time to go off the drugs. You may need to seek professional help with this or use the methods described below to wean. The withdrawal symptoms of recreational drugs are a little bit worse withdrawal symptoms of the others. Seek professional help with weaning from recreational drugs.

Next, wean from excessive alcohol. It helps to wean slowly. Determine how many drinks you take in a day. The first week, drink half that amount each day. The second week, half again, the third week, either be down to one drink, or quit cold turkey. It is okay to drink one or two drinks a day if your physician says you can.

Likewise, try to break the other bad habits, smoking, caffeine, and junk food. Whether or not you stop all of the bad habits, it is up to you, but the one that must be broken for sure is the junk food habit, in order to make either the clean eating diet or the belly fat diet a success. Junk food habits can be broken at the same time you start the diet, however sugar is very addictive and your body will crave this food, wanting more of it. If you stop the junk without weaning, you will have intense moments of craving and a strong desire to cave in. Rather than go through this, why not start the diet while you wean?

Assess how much junk you eat in one day. Start by slashing that in half, and replace the other half with a nutritious snack. Eat this way for a week. Then continue, the 2nd week, slash the junk in half again, replacing the junk with a nutritious snack. Slash the junk consumption in half again the third week, replacing again with nutritious food. By the third week you should be on so little junk food you should have very little issues with stopping it completely by the fourth week.

Since you are wanting a low fat diet to help get rid of excessive weight and fat, let us talk about exercise.

Exercise will take you further faster with the diet and the losing of the weight than if you just did the diet alone. Your body's metabolism will speed up if you exercise, helping it to burn the fat and calories faster. Because exercising speeds the metabolism, you will want to get up and exercise to burn the energy. Exercise does not need to be complicated. You do not have to join a gym and work out with a personal trainer. You can exercise right from your home, or go to a park. Just walking for a half an hour at a time will do your body a lot of good. The key to success with exercising is to spend at least half an hour at a time being physically active, every other day at minimum. That is just three days a week for an effective way to help the low fat diet be a bigger success.

Disclaimer: The information contained within this book is just that, for information purposes only. We are not medical professionals, but we do advise you seek the counsel of your health care provider before starting any new diet or exercise routine. You especially need their direction if you are going to try to break free from the bad habits you may have started. Once your health care provider gives you the go ahead, read through this book again and start planning your meals.

The two diet plans within this book are very similar. If

you are weaning from junk food, you may want to include the clean eating diet during the weaning period. Once you are weaned from the junk food, go on the belly fat diet and make a goal to stick with it. But if you "cheat" and eat something junky, do not be upset with yourself. Just get back to the diet with the next meal and move on to losing the fat.

Section 1: Clean Eating

Have you ever wished that someone would write a cookbook that gives just the facts? All diets put an emphasis on their particular type of foods and how they are beneficial, but many real factors are often eliminated, in order to promote a specific diet. Look no further. The Clean Cook Book is designed to present not only facts about the food you eat, but give you real choices in giving your body the cleanest foods possible, and obtainable. Learn how flour, sugar, bread, and milk, are not always what they appear, and can contribute to a decrease in the function of your system.

In addition, discover how processed and genetically modified products have no real nutrition in the anatomy of humans, but were simply created to preserve and extend shelf life. Once you realize how one, two, or all of these foodstuffs can play a part in limiting a long and fruitful life, the real fun begins. Recipes that are unique, tasty, and great for your body, are categorized and presented with detailed instructions. Isn't it time that you made a conscious decision about what is healthy and what is not? Gather the information, use the list of substitutes, and know that you are doing all that you can to offer your body the nutrients it requires.

Let's Get Real

Fresh fruits and vegetables, lean meats, seafood and fiber-rich grains, all sound like a great start to eating healthy. But, let's be realistic. Who has the resources, money and time to track down all of these nutritious foods on a daily basis? Wouldn't we all love to live next door to a fresh market that could provide us with all the foods that diets insist that we need? The fact is, most of us try to pick up fresh items, when available and not too pricey, but the rest of the time, it's canned foods and cheap boxed pastas. Learn how to use what is available and to take advantage of those fresh foods when you can. Also, discover 10 healthy tips, in this informative book, for a cleaner way of eating.

Mind Controlling Foods

No, this is not a weird, conspiracy theory as to why we cannot lose weight. Nor is it a way to train your mind into being submissive over sweets and breads. It is simply an explanation as to how the human anatomy works. No one can argue the fact that your mind controls your hunger, or that it tells you what is tasty and what is rotten. There are certain chemicals that cause the brain to search for what the body needs. You hear a lot about hormones today and this is because hormones is the control center that tells your mind exactly what your body needs. Become introduced to these chemicals, how they interact with the brain, and why fad diets never seem to work.

Foods that Send Negative Messages

Some people have allergies that prevent them from enjoying certain foods. Shell fish, peanuts and milk are good examples of products that can have negative reactions to certain individuals. It does not take very long for a person with food allergies, to realize that they have to live without food that causes them misery.

In a world where processed foods have become a way of life, it can be difficult to steer clear of all products that have been chemically altered. In some cases, processed foods are actually good for you. Take milk, for instance. Through pasteurizing, dangerous bacteria is eliminated for safe consumption. However, most foods use processing for convenience. Knowing the difference between safety and convenience, when shopping, will help you to make wise meal choices.

Once you know what the real facts are about the foods you eat, a plan can be put into action. A 5-day planner is also included to get you on the right track to feeling better, living longer, and yes, even losing weight. Be prepared to get inspired, get reconnected with your body's needs, and enjoy terrific meals from a book filled with tantalizing foods. Breakfast, lunch, dinner, snacks, and beverages, will taste better, give you more energy, lose those last impossible 10 pounds, and not crimp your budget, After a while, heavily processed foods will begin to taste like cardboard, just like they do to your body.

Chapter 1: The Clean Diet

There are several renditions of clean dieting on the book shelves today. Some are written by physicians, experts in nutrition or personal trainers. Cleansing programs, cutting out junk foods, and eliminating processed foods, are a few of the diets that are promoted. While all of these suggestions have merit, weaving these solutions into one's daily life can be a bit uncomfortable. There should be nothing complex or restraining about a new way of living with food. If your body is deprived of certain addictions, food will be foremost on your brain, and that is no fun.

Most of us know that fresh vegetables, fruit and lean meats are good for us. But our brains tell us that potato chips and chocolate cake are too good to let go. The whole point of a clean diet is to wean your food desires off of garbage, that do nothing but pollute your system. Your entire life has probably evolved around eating unhealthy foods and stopping cold turkey, doesn't work.

Wants and Needs

Remember when microwave ovens or cell phones were first introduced? These are items that clearly define the difference between wants and needs. Ask yourself if either one of these are absolutely necessary to live a full and fruitful life. Of course they aren't, but marketing and peer pressure have set the tone by mixing up wants and needs. Have you ever had a craving for something natural, like an apple, fresh green beans or a melon? This is your body trying to signal your brain that your body is hungry! This is not a want, but a need that has been ignored for way too long.

As we age, our taste in foods change. This is not from the aging process but from an addiction to fast food, chemicals used in processed items, and a slower metabolism that wants some form of comfort. Perhaps you have developed a case of indigestion from certain foods, or find that those desserts that you once loved, make you groggy. Everything is a signal from our bodies that they need nutrition and this is their reminder that is not going to go away. Many people have lost their sense of taste from not eating vitamin-enriched vegetables and fruits. Deep fried foods is one of the worst culprits for robbing your taste buds of flavor. You are feeding your body refined flour that has been dipped in reused vegetable oil. What is inside the coating becomes irrelevant, compared to the fat that beats any type of nutrition to your stomach.

Your taste in foods has not really changed. What has changed, is your body's unwillingness to tolerate being fed foods that clog arteries, eat away at stomach and colon linings, and raise havoc on your hormones and immune system. Once you begin cutting back on chemically-laced foods, you will notice how much better a chicken breast tastes, over a rare steak, or strawberries over chocolate cake. These are signals that your body has had enough abuse and wants to repair itself. It is never too late to take that first step toward healthy eating. You will find yourself actually enjoying a meal, with no repercussions of stomach pain, headaches, being listless, or possibly creating food allergies.

Keep your Freedom of Food

Some popular diets use ingredients that sound foreign to you, because they are. Finding the right blends of seasonings and herbs to cover the taste of tofu, can be a real adventure. The recipes that you are about to find in this book, are nothing out of the ordinary. In fact, some of the recipes that you find, may resemble old fashioned dishes that you used to find at family reunions. Now that is something to look forward to.

Chapter 2: Benefits of Clean Eating

We have been taught that clean, healthy eating is important. Eating three meals a day, drinking plenty of liquids, and balancing the five food groups, are essential to a body's growth and maintenance. However, no one teaches us the truth about how some of our food has been modified and chemically treated, for the sake of higher profits. More grain per acre, more weight per package with fillers, and more additives for longer shelf life, have taken these once nutritional-based foods and replaced them with damaging chemicals. The FDA will tell you that in small amounts, these additives are not harmful, but over an extended period of time, can damage the body. Here are a few facts of how our bodies react to unnatural presences.

Balances Hormones

Leptin is a hormone that opens or closes the door on when we feel hungry. A high level of Leptin will take food from stored fat before signaling the body to ask for food. A low level of Leptin will signal a hunger that needs to be fed. An obese person, normally has a high level of Leptin, which means that they should not be hungry, due to all the stored fat. However, when you constantly feed your body processed and GMO products, the body does not recognize nutrition, and screams to be fed. The fat is just that, fat. No vitamins or nutrition to feed off of. As far as your system is concerned, there is nothing in those fat cells but worthless cardboard. So the overweight person will continue to eat, trying to repair a hunger that is never satisfied.

Ghrelin is often referred to as the 'feel good hormone', because it delivers a message to the brain. Do you want a salad or chocolate cake? Too much ghrelin tells the brain that chocolate cake is best, while low levels of ghrelin, sees little difference between the two choices. The medical community is convinced that by blocking ghrelin, obesity can be controlled. A drug to counteract this, is now in the works. Once again, the body is confused as to what to do with foods that offer no nutrient value, and is throwing the hormone off balance. Instead of developing a new drug that blocks these two vital hormones, wouldn't it be better to create a healthy environment for them?

What is Wrong with White Flour and Refined Sugar?

It seems that white flour is used in almost everything we eat. Pasta, bread, cereal and crackers, use white flour to help hold a nice form and texture. Most people do not really understand what white flour really is. Made from multiple grains, like wheat, rice and corn, it takes quite a bit of processing to turn into a powdery consistency. During this process, vitamins are removed, chemicals and preservatives are added, plus a little dye to make the nice white color. There is nothing of nutritional value in white flour, but plenty to be afraid of.

Refined sugar is an important carbohydrate in our lives and a little bit can actually be healthy. However, we no longer have any control over what products contain sugar and what products do not. Look at any package in your grocery store. If you see an ingredient with a -ose on the end of a word, it contains some form of sugar. Each teaspoon of sugar you use, equals 15 calories and 4 grams of carbs. That may not sound like a lot, but add to that the 50 carbs that your bottle of tea had in it, and you are in sugar shock. Artificial sweeteners are nothing more than toxic chemicals that mimic sugar, but your body knows the difference. Making your own meals with real sugar, or the choices shown in the next chapter, can save you from indulging in sugar, and not even knowing it.

Our bodies were specifically designed to eat the foods that have been made available to us. Meat, milk and eggs for protein, vegetables and fruit for vitamins, and grain for fiber. However, when companies play with Mother Nature, our human anatomy goes into danger-mode. A clean diet will put your system back on track and bring relief to a body that has been battling these unknown substances for years.

Chapter 3: Alternative Food Types

You can stay within the realm of healthy foods without going totally vegan or organic in your cooking. There are many alternatives that can be used in the place of genetically modified foods, such as bleached flour or refined sugar. Here are some lists of alternative choices that you can keep in your kitchen cupboards.

Flour (without Gluten)

buckwheat flour
brown rice flour
millet flour
quinoa flour
sorghum flour
oat flour
tapioca flour
white rice flour
arrowroot flour
coconut flour

Sugar (without preservatives)

Cactus powder
Organic Palm sugar
Stevia
Sucanat
Dextrose
Evaporated coconut palm sugar
Sorbitol
Agave powder
Honey
Real maple syrup

There are other natural and organic products to choose from but these are the most common. Almost everything we consume today, is made out of bleached flour and refined sugar. By simply switching to a healthier form of flour and sugar, in your meal preparation, you will notice a dramatic difference in the way you feel.

Natural Home Made Mayonnaise

Another type of food that is preservative-laced, is a jar of mayonnaise or salad dressing. Mayonnaise is simply eggs and oil mixed together. However, doesn't it strike you as odd, that a jar of mayonnaise or salad dressing, can last anywhere from 3 months to 1 year? There are tons of preservatives here. Make your own mayonnaise that will taste better, be totally fresh, and not contain one foreign chemical. This recipe makes 2 cups, will last for 5 days, refrigerated, and only takes 5 minutes to make.

Ingredients

2 egg yolks
1 whole egg
1 TBSP fresh lemon juice
½ tsp salt
1/8 tsp white pepper
2 cups pure olive oil

Instructions

Using a blender, place egg, egg yolks, lemon juice, salt and pepper inside. Blend until smooth, about 10 to 15 seconds.

Place the olive oil in a cup so you can add in small streams. Turn the blender on the lowest speed and slowly add the oil in droplets, about 1/8 of a cup. Turn off the blender and wait 30 seconds.

The reason for this is so the chemical reaction of the lemon juice and egg yolks will have a chance to stabilize.

Otherwise, the two will not merge and you will have a separation of oil and eggs.
Continue this process until your ingredients become thick and creamy.

Spoon into an airtight jar and keep refrigerated.

Chapter 4: Tips for Eating Clean and Healthy

Clean eating doesn't have to involve living like a survivalist and never buying anything from the grocery. That would not be very practical. From time to time, you are going to be in a pinch for money, or time, and convenience foods just have to do. Here are some tips to eat as clean as possible, without falling completely off of the wagon.

Wash all liquid off of vegetables and fruits that are packed in a can.

Buy frozen vegetables and fruit instead of canned.

Choose white basmati rice over plain milled white rice.

Whole grain bread has not been refined while whole wheat bread, has.

Real butter is better for you than margarine. Use olive oil or canola oil instead of vegetable oil.

Use sea salt instead of refined salt.

Save fresh vegetable scraps to use as stock for soups.

Select American or Canadian albacore tuna over chunk or canned light tuna.

Watch out for terms, such as fruit flavored drinks, that are sugar water.

Eat dark chocolate as opposed to milk chocolate.

These tips are not designed to give you permission to indulge on tons of real butter or dark chocolate, but to give you better eating options, how to use your shopping dollars wisely, and to move toward a clean diet, naturally.

Chapter 5: 5-Day Sample Planner for Day to Day Meals

Wanting to cook right, for your family, is not always easy. Time seems to run thin and before you know it, you're sitting in line at a fast food restaurant. By making a plan, shopping for the right foods, and convincing yourself that nothing is more important than health, you will find the time to reward your body for the stress and abuse that it has endured. Here is a sample of a day to day planner to help get started on how to create a schedule that will work. You will know what needs to be done in advance and not feel so rushed when meal time rolls around.

Monday

Breakfast: Granola cereal with milk and a banana, hot green tea or coffee

Lunch: Albacore tuna pita, cheese slices, sliced apple, carrot sticks, fruit   smoothie

Snack: Granola mix

Dinner: Beef asparagus stir-fry, side salad and fresh lemonade

Tuesday

Breakfast: Apple ring pancakes with maple syrup, hot green tea or coffee

Lunch: Greens and berries super salad, baked tostados, fruit smoothie

Snack: Celery sticks with peanut butter

Dinner: Homemade tacos, angel food cake with sliced strawberries, lime   spritzer

Wednesday

Breakfast: Granola cereal and banana bread, hot green tea or coffee

Lunch: Reuben sandwich, baked chips, cucumber slices, fruit smoothie

Snack: Dark chocolate bar

Dinner: Fish fillets, stuffed zucchini boats, banana bread,

fresh lemonade

Thursday

Breakfast: Scrambled eggs, muffins, fresh squeezed orange juice

Lunch: Egg salad on whole-grain bread, chicken soup, sliced tomatoes , green tea

Snack: Granola mix

Dinner: Oven chili, cornbread, veggie platter with dip, milk shake

Friday

Breakfast: Oatmeal with raisins and almonds, orange sections, toast, hot green tea or coffee

Lunch: Salmon with cucumber salsa, side salad, tapioca pudding, green tea

Snack: Apple and cheese slices

Dinner: Grilled jerk chicken, spring pea-cheddar salad, chocolate cake, fruit smoothie

You can use this planner for your first week, using the delicious recipes that follow, or create one of your own. The idea is to think ahead and have a plan in your mind. Then, watch how simple it is for everything to fall into place.

Chapter 6: Breakfast Recipes

Breakfast Fiesta

Makes 2 Servings

Create Mexican colors, without the south-of-the border taste. This attractive, filling egg dish has all the makings for an energized morning. Plenty of protein with high vitamins and minerals, will keep you going for hours.

INGREDIENTS:

1 egg yolk
6 egg whites
½ tsp oregano, dried
½ tsp paprika
1 tsp sunflower oil
2 cups cubed whole-grain bread
1 zucchini, sliced julienne
1 minced red bell pepper
1 chopped tomato

INSTRUCTIONS:

Place yolk, egg whites, oregano and paprika in a medium-sized bowl. Whisk together and set aside.

Warm the sunflower oil in a large skillet to high heat. Saute the bread, pepper, zucchini and tomato, constantly stirring. After about 3 minutes, or when vegetables begin to brown, pour the egg mixture, in a circle, over the top.

Continue stirring until the eggs are cooked through. Turn onto a platter and serve.

Rise and Shine Banana Bread

Makes 8 Servings

Dessert for breakfast? You bet, but without the unhealthy preservatives and heavy fats of donuts. Serve up with a mixture of melon or berries and feel the difference in your morning. You won't be sluggish or tired and will be full of natural metabolism to start the day.

INGREDIENTS:

4 smashed, ripe bananas
1/3 cup butter, melted
1 cup natural sugar substitute
1 egg, beaten
1 tsp vanilla
1 tsp baking soda
1 ½ cups natural flour
Canola oil spray

INSTRUCTIONS:

Heat oven to 350 degrees F.

Using a large mixing bowl, combine the bananas and

butter and mix. Add the egg, sugar, vanilla and baking soda. Mix well.

Add the flour in 4 sections, stirring well between each batch.

Pour the mixture into a loaf pan that has been lightly sprayed with canola oil.

Bake in oven for 50-60 minutes. Remove from oven and cool on a rack.

Sweet and Zesty Pancake Apple Rings

Makes 4 Servings

Pancakes are tempting, and fattening, when the wrong ingredients are used. Never let this stop you from enjoying this fruity rendition of zesty apple rings. And by all means, pass the real maple syrup.

INGREDIENTS:

1 cup flour natural flour
1 TBSP sugar substitute
2 tsp baking powder
¼ tsp sea salt
½ tsp lemon peel
½ tsp cinnamon
1 egg, beaten
1 cup milk
2 TBSP canola oil
2 apples, pared, cored and sliced 1/2-inch thick

INSTRUCTIONS:

In a medium-sized bowl, combine flour, sugar substitute, baking powder, salt, lemon peel and cinnamon. Blend well. Stir in the egg, milk, and oil.

Add 1 TBSP butter to a large skillet and melt over medium heat.

Using a pair of tongs, dip each apple slice in the batter and add to skillet. Make sure not to overlap so each battered apple can be browned completely. Flip over to brown the other side. Remove as completed and repeat until all apples have been cooked. You may have to add additional butter to your skillet between batches.

Healthy Granola Breakfast Cereal

Makes 8 Servings

Stay away from expensive, sugar-laced breakfast cereals that offer little nutrient value by making your own fresh cereal that can be stored for the entire week. This granola cereal version can be weaved with different dried fruits, depending on your taste.

INGREDIENTS:

3 ½ cups natural rolled oats
¼ cup raw sunflower seeds, without the shell
½ cup almonds
½ cup raw coconut flakes
1 cup raisins
1 cup dried cranberries
2 tsp cinnamon
2 TBSP honey
1 tsp sea salt
¼ cup sugar substitute
1 TBSP real maple syrup
¼ cup canola oil
2 tsp vanilla

INSTRUCTIONS:

Heat oven to 375 degrees F.

Use a large rimmed baking sheet and place a layer of aluminum foil on the surface.

In a large mixing bowl, combine all dry ingredients (except the raisins and cranberries) and mix. Drizzle with the liquids and turn onto the baking sheet.

Place in the oven for 10 minutes. Remove and toss the mixture. Repeat every 10 minutes for 30 minutes. Remove and cool.

Add raisins and cranberries, mix, and place in an air-tight container.

Springtime Baked Omelet

Makes 8 Servings

Use vegetables from the garden, or road side stand, in selecting the freshest produce available for this robust springtime morning meal. The sweet potatoes will bring an intriguing rich flavor when mixed with the other succulent veggies. Plenty of vitamins, minerals and protein will start off your day with a new outlook.

INGREDIENTS:

2 sweet potatoes
¼ cup chopped onion
1 cup shredded Cheddar cheese
1 cup zucchini, sliced thin
6 eggs
1 cup milk
¼ cup substitute flour
½ tsp sea salt
1/8 tsp ground black pepper
1 chopped tomato

INSTRUCTIONS:

Warm oven to 400 degrees F. Using spray Canola oil,

coat the interior of a deep dish baking pan.

Peel, wash and slice the sweet potatoes. Layer in the pan, along with the chopped onion. Sprinkle the cheese on top of the potatoes and onion. Arrange the zucchini slices atop the cheese.

In a large mixing bowl, combine eggs, milk, flour, pepper and sea salt and blend with a whisk or a mixer. Pour the mixture over the layered vegetables.

Bake for 30-40 minutes, or until the center is set. Remove and top with chopped tomatoes. Slice and serve.

Chapter 7: Quick and Easy Lunches

Reuben Supreme Sandwich

Makes 1 Serving

If you have ever worked or lived close to a Deli, you may have been fortunate enough to feast on a Reuben sandwich. Although this meaty, tart luncheon special is well over 100 years old, many have never tried it. Even if you are not a big fan of rye bread, this could turn into a lunchtime favorite for curbing your hunger.

INGREDIENTS:

2 slices thinly cut turkey breast
¼ cup fresh sauerkraut
1 Mozzarella cheese slice
2 slices dill whole-grain rye bread
2 TBSP low-fat Thousand Island dressing
1 TBSP mustard

INSTRUCTIONS:

Spread the Thousand Island dressing on 1 slice of rye bread. Stack with the turkey slices, sauerkraut and Mozzarella cheese.

Spray a skillet with Canola oil and turn to medium heat. Place the top layer of bread on top of the ingredients, making a sandwich. Toast both sides of the bread until lightly toasted. If the Mozzarella cheese is not completely melted, but the bread is toasted nicely, remove from pan and cover the sandwich with a paper towel and place in the microwave for 30-50 seconds.

Creamy Albacore Pita

Makes 4 Servings

Tuna salad doesn't have to be boring and tasteless. By using healthy vegetables, your homemade mayonnaise, and whole-grain pita pockets, lunchtime becomes a time to enjoy. You can also use plain nonfat yogurt in the place of mayonnaise.

INGREDIENTS:

1- 6 ½ ounce can water-packed albacore tuna
2 stalks celery, chopped fine
2 green onions, sliced thin
1 TBSP fresh dill
½ cup homemade mayonnaise or nonfat plain yogurt
2 tsp mustard
¼ tsp celery seed
4 whole-grain pita pockets
Lettuce leaves
Sliced tomato

INSTRUCTIONS:

Drain the albacore tuna well. Flake with a fork and add celery, green onion, and dill. Stir in mayo or yogurt, mustard, and celery seed.

Place lettuce leaves and tomato inside pita before spooning the tuna inside.

Touch of Italy Cheese Quesadillas

Makes 8 servings

Plan the perfect luncheon with friends and impress them with your low-calorie, melt-in-your-mouth Italian treats that make a meal. Borrowing an idea from the Spanish culture and stuffing with Italian flavors, will make you a hit for the day.

INGREDIENTS:

8- 7 inch whole-grain flour tortillas
1 fresh garlic clove, pressed
1/3 cup black olives, sliced
3 sliced plum tomatoes
¼ cup fresh basil
1 cups shredded Mozzarella cheese
½ cup Feta cheese, crumbled
olive oil

INSTRUCTIONS:

Turn on oven to 425 degrees F. Place 4 tortillas on a round pizza pie pan. Press garlic cloves into surface. Spread ¼ cup Mozzarella cheese on the tortillas.

Lay tomatoes on top of the cheese. Next, place olives around the mixture. Sprinkle with the basil leaves. Crumble the Feta cheese on top.

Put a whole-grain flour tortilla on top of each prepared tortilla and spray the top with olive oil. Bake for 8-10 minutes. Remove and layer the remaining Mozzarella cheese on top of the four sandwiched tortillas. Return to oven until cheese has melted. Remove, cool and cut into wedges.

Greens and Berries Super Salad

Makes 8 Servings

Sometimes a salad just sounds good. However, it does not take long for lettuce and low-fat dressing to lose its appeal. A combination of greens and berries is never boring. You will also find that no dressing is necessary, because every bite will be sweet and flavorful. Keep your ingredients separated and have ready to throw 1-2 servings together in an instant.

INGREDIENTS:

½ head romaine lettuce
½ head iceberg lettuce
1 sliced pear
1 orange
12 sliced strawberries
2 kiwi, sliced
4 fresh mushrooms, sliced
3 TBSP Romano cheese
2 TBSP Parmesan cheese
1 TBSP olive oil, mixed with basil and parsley

INSTRUCTIONS:

In a large salad bowl, tear the lettuce into bite-sized pieces.

Cut the orange into 4 sections and squeeze the juice from 2 of these into a cup. Chop up the other 2 sections and add to greens. Add the pear, strawberries, kiwi, and mushrooms.

Toss all. Pour the orange juice overall then sprinkle the cheeses on top. Finish with a touch of seasoned olive oil.

Marinated Salmon with Cucumber Salsa

Makes 4 Servings

Salmon takes on a delightful flavor when drenched in a fresh cucumber-based salsa. Make ahead of time and store in the refrigerator. The different flavors will be a welcome treat in the middle of the day.

INGREDIENTS:

4 fresh or frozen salmon fillets

Marinade:

2 TBSP olive oil
1 TBSP cilantro
1 TBSP ground ginger root
¼ teaspoon sea salt
¼ teaspoon black pepper

Salsa:

1 cup chopped cucumber
¼ cup chopped red onion
¼ cup chopped red bell pepper
1 jalapeno pepper, seeded and chopped

1 pressed garlic clove
3 TBSP rice vinegar
2 TBSP olive oil
¼ teaspoon sugar substitute
1/8 teaspoon sea salt

INSTRUCTIONS:

For marinade, combine ingredients in a small bowl and blend.

Place salmon fillets in an air tight plastic bag. Pour the marinade over the fillets and seal. Place in refrigerator and allow to marinade for 1 hour.

For salsa, press garlic into a medium-sized bowl. Add vinegar, oil, sugar and salt. Mix well. Add all vegetables and toss. Put aside.

Heat oven to 400 degrees F.

Remove salmon from marinade and place on a flat baking dish. Bake for 15-20 minutes, or until salmon flakes easily with a fork. Remove from oven and serve with marinade.

Chapter 8: Main Meal Recipes

Beef Asparagus Stir-Fry

Makes 4 Servings

Get out the wok and create a dinner with sides included. This is where your saved chicken or vegetable stock will come in handy in adding a rich taste to sweet, young asparagus and beef. This can also be a great time to test out quinoa rice, known for a slightly strong flavor, or serve with wild whole-grain rice and soup or salad.

INGREDIENTS:

1 pound beef flank steak
2 TBSP soy sauce
4 TBSP olive oil or Canola oil
1 TBSP cornstarch
12 fresh, young asparagus spears
1 teaspoon sugar substitute
4 TBSP chicken or vegetable stock liquid

INSTRUCTIONS:

Cut the flank steak into thin strips, slicing against the grain. In a small bowl, combine soy sauce and 1 tablespoon oil. Drizzle this mixture over the steak strips. Allow to marinade while preparing the asparagus.

Cut the asparagus spears diagonally in 1-inch pieces and drop into a saucepan of boiling water. Simmer for 2 minutes, then drain.

In the wok, heat 3 tablespoons oil until it begins to sizzle. Sprinkle the sugar substitute over the oil. Add the beef cuts and stir for 1 minute. Add the asparagus pieces and stir for an additional minute. Pour the broth overall and stir for 1 more minute.

Turn onto platter and serve with rice or quinoa.

Home Made Beef Tacos with Salsa

Makes 6 Servings

Instead of buying packages of taco seasoning on taco night, use a more nutritional homemade mix with fresh ingredients that will leave you feeling filled and refreshed. Packaged seasonings contain massive amounts of salt, sugar, dyes and chemicals. Nothing that your body wants or needs.

INGREDIENTS:

Taco seasoning and fixings:

1 pound lean ground beef
1 finely chopped garlic clove
½ teaspoon sea salt
1 TBSP vinegar
1 TBSP chili powder
1 TBSP hot pepper sauce
½ teaspoon cornstarch
¼ to ½ cup water
6 soft or hard taco shells
lettuce, shredded
tomatoes, diced
shredded cheddar cheese

diced onion

Seasoned tomato salsa:

3 tomatoes, peeled and diced
½ red onion, chopped
1 jalapeno pepper, seeded and chopped
1 Serrano chili pepper, seeded and diced
1 lime
½ cup diced cilantro

INSTRUCTIONS:

Make the salsa first so it has time to absorb all the flavors.

Combine the tomatoes, onion, peppers and cilantro in a medium-sized bowl. Toss well. Cut the lime in quarters and squeeze the juice into the mix. Depending on your taste, you may only wish to use ¼ to ½ lime.

In a small bowl, combine the clove, sea salt, vinegar, chili powder, pepper sauce and cornstarch. Mix well and set aside.

Use a medium to large skillet and brown the hamburger. Pour off the grease. Add the taco seasonings, along with enough water to keep moist. Stir over medium heat until the desired consistency occurs.

Scoop into taco shells, dress with lettuce, tomatoes, cheese and onions, and pass the salsa.

Crispy Fish Fillets with Lemon Dip

Makes 4 Servings

It is easy to tire of bland baked fish, especially without tartar sauce. Use this recipe to fry up a catch of walleye, haddock or pollock and experience the luscious flavors of fresh fish, lemon and dill. The secret is in the crumbs, made from baked chips that you once thought had little taste.

INGREDIENTS:

4 fish fillets
2 ounces baked chips (veggie, Lays, Pringles)
2 TBSP canola oil
½ cup homemade mayonnaise
3 TBSP fresh chopped dill
2 teaspoons grated lemon peel
¼ teaspoon pepper

INSTRUCTIONS:

Place baked chips in a large freezer zip-lock bag and roll until crumbly. Spread out on a piece of flat waxed paper. Drag the fillets through the crumbs until coated on both sides.

In a small bowl, mix the mayonnaise, dill, lemon peel and pepper. Set aside as the dip.

In a large skillet, pour 1 tablespoon oil and turn on medium heat. Cook 2 pieces of fish at a time, so as not to crowd, carefully turning over after 3-4 minutes. Remove and repeat with remaining fillets.

Thick and Chunky Oven Chili

Makes 12 Servings

There is nothing more satisfying than a big bowl of hearty beef chili. By using natural ingredients, you can keep this dish as nutritional as a meal that offers little taste. Rich seasonings surrounding chunks of stew meat, will hit the spot and fill you quickly. Great for warming up as leftovers.

INGREDIENTS:

3 pounds beef roast or stew meat
4 pressed garlic cloves
2 TBSP chili powder
1 ½ teaspoons dried oregano leaves
¾ teaspoon cumin
¼ teaspoon sea salt
¼ teaspoon ground black pepper
2 cups chopped onions
2 cups chopped green bell pepper
6 peeled fresh tomatoes
1 pound black, pinto, or kidney beans, cooked
16 ounces tomato sauce

INSTRUCTIONS:

Heat oven to 350 degrees F.

Cut meat into ½ inch cubes and place in a large mixing bowl. Press garlic into meat. Add chili powder, oregano leaves, cumin, salt and pepper, and toss.

Pour into a deep baking dish with lid. Add onions, pepper, tomatoes sauce and beans. Mix lightly and cover.

Bake for 2 hours and remove. Skim off the fat from the top and discard. Return to oven for another 30 minutes, or until meat is tender. Remove from oven and skim off any remaining grease. Stir and serve.

Savory Scallops with Zesty Spinach

Makes 4 Servings

Calling seafood lovers everywhere. Nothing says taste, like buttery scallops and lemon coated veggies. Try this intriguing dish that will awaken your taste buds and make you feel as if a $100 meal was just prepared. Sea scallops can be an extravagant treat, so save for a very special occasion.

INGREDIENTS:

2 pounds or about 26 sea scallops
¼ teaspoon sea salt
¼ teaspoon pepper
3 TBSP butter
1 clove garlic, minced
10 ounces baby spinach
1 ½ TBSP fresh lemon juice
2 TBSP fresh chopped chives
2 teaspoons grated lemon peel

INSTRUCTIONS:

Using a large skillet, melt one tablespoon butter over medium heat. Add garlic and stir until fragrant.

Approximately 30 seconds. Add spinach and stir until it becomes wilted. Remove spinach and garlic to a platter and cover to keep warm.

With a paper towel, wipe out the skillet and place back on the stove over medium heat. Melt 2 tablespoons butter and wait for it to start sizzling. Add one-half scallops, seasoning with sea salt and pepper. Cook until browned on both sides and opaque. Remove and repeat with second batch of scallops. Cover all cooked scallops with foil to keep warm.

Turn off stove and add lemon juice to butter drippings. Stir slightly and add chives and lemon peel.

Turn the spinach onto a platter and make a bed for the scallops. Carefully spoon the scallops onto the spinach and drizzle with the butter, lemon drippings.

No Problem Grilled Jerk Chicken

Makes 8 Servings

Jamaica is famous for creating jerk chicken out of only fresh ingredients. While you can find imitation products in seasoning packets, nothing compares to the distinct taste of making your own sauce. Here is an incredible recipe that comes very close to the unforgettable jerk chicken of the Caribbean.

INGREDIENTS:

4 chicken breasts
4 chicken legs
4 chicken thighs
3 chopped scallions
1 onion, chopped
3 pressed garlic cloves
4 chili peppers, seeded and chopped
¼ cup fresh lime juice
2 TBSP soy sauce
3 TBSP olive oil
¾ teaspoon sea salt
1 TBSP brown sugar, packed
¾ teaspoon fresh nutmeg, grated
2 teaspoons allspice

1 teaspoon black pepper
1 TBSP fresh thyme
½ teaspoon cinnamon

INSTRUCTIONS:

Place all ingredients (except chicken pieces) in a blender and blend.

Use 2 gallon-sized zip-lock bags and place all chicken pieces, equally, inside. Pour the marinade evenly over the chicken and close, removing most of the air. Allow to marinade overnight in the refrigerator, turning over a couple of times.

Prepare the grill by getting the coals hot. Lightly grease the rack and grill each chicken piece over the hottest portion of the grill for 3-4 minutes for each side. After they are well-seared, move to the side where the coals are not directly under the chicken pieces and cover with a lid or aluminum foil for at least 30 minutes, or until fully cooked throughout.

Chapter 9: Side Dishes

Cauliflower Fanfare

Makes 6 Servings

Cauliflower becomes more than just a crunchy vegetable when you outfit it with colorful additions and flavors. A unique zesty dressing makes this side dish perfect for picnics or casual dinners.

INGREDIENTS:

1 TBSP onion, chopped
1 garlic clove, minced
1 TBSP olive oil
2 TBSP Italian low-fat salad dressing
3 cups bite-sized cauliflowers
2 TBSP chopped green pepper
1 cup cherry tomatoes, halved
¼ teaspoon crushed fresh basil
¼ cup water

INSTRUCTIONS:

Using a saucepan, sauté the onion and garlic in the 1 TBSP olive oil. Add water and simmer for 7-10 minutes. Remove from heat and add the basil and salad dressing. Stir until well blended and set aside to cool.

In a large salad bowl, combine the cauliflowers, green pepper and tomatoes.

Pour the sauce over the vegetables and toss.

Quinoa Corn Salad

Makes 8 Servings

If you are unfamiliar with quinoa, you owe it to yourself to try. Often used as a replacement for grains, quinoa is actually a vegetable with a unique flavor. You will never find as many vitamins and anti-oxidants than in these little beans. Mixed with other beans, corn, and peppers, the taste is welcoming and may become a favorite of yours.

INGREDIENTS:

2 cups quinoa
¼ cup olive oil
1 teaspoon ground cumin
3 cups fresh cooked corn
1 cup black beans
1 red bell pepper, diced
1 orange bell pepper, diced
1 jalapeno pepper, seeded and chopped
1 cup cilantro, chopped
1 lime
¼ teaspoon red pepper flakes

INSTRUCTIONS:

Rinse and drain quinoa in a strainer. Using a medium saucepan, boil 4 cups of water and add the quinoa all at once. When the water starts to boil again, reduce heat, cover with lid and let simmer for 10 to 15 minutes, or until all the water has been absorbed. Remove from heat and allow to cool.

Use a small bowl to make the dressing. Add the olive oil, cumin and pepper flakes. Cut the lime in half and squeeze the juice into the mixture. Whisk well and set aside.

Using a large salad bowl, add corn, beans, bell peppers, cilantro and jalapeno. Add the cooled quinoa and stir. Drizzle the dressing over all, mix and serve.

Stuffed Zucchini Boats

Makes 4 Servings

Use the outer shell of your zucchini for a great display of this tasty vegetable, plus eggs, cheese and tomatoes. Be warned, however. The taste can be addictive and you will find your family asking for stuffed boats, regularly.

INGREDIENTS:

4 medium-sized zucchini squash
1 large tomato
3 beaten eggs
½ cup shredded American cheese
2 TBSP butter
½ cup water
1/8 teaspoon sea salt

INSTRUCTIONS:

Cut each zucchini in half, long-ways. With a spoon, scoop out the veggie meat, leaving a ¼ inches all the way around the shell. Take the veggie meat and pulp to make 1 cup. Set aside.

Take a large skillet and place the zucchini shells face

down in the skillet. Add water and cover. Turn on heat to medium and simmer, just until boats are tender, 5-6 minutes. Remove from stove, drain off water, and turn zucchini face side up in the same skillet. Sprinkle with sea salt.

Using a separate medium-sized skillet, cook the zucchini pump and tomato in the butter about 3 minutes, or until squash is tender. Add eggs, a sprinkle of sea salt, and pepper. Cook until everything is set, using a spatula to stir, like making scrambled eggs.

Spoon the mixture into each zucchini boat and top with cheese. Cover and heat until the cheese is melted.

Sassy Apricots and Sweet Potatoes

Makes 4 Servings

It is a fact that all of the daily health requirements are contained in a single sweet potato. If you could learn to live on this one vegetable, you would receive all of the essential vitamins and minerals that your body needs. Here is an unusual dish, using sweet potatoes, that could just put you in the mood for this great vegetable, more often.

INGREDIENTS:

1 cup dried apricots
2 ½ cups sweet potatoes
¾ cup orange juice
½ cup water
3 TBSP brown sugar
2 TBSP honey
2 TBSP butter
½ cup walnut halves

INSTRUCTIONS:

Heat oven to 375 degrees F.

Peel, cut and sweet potatoes into chunks. Place in a baking dish and cook until tender.

In a saucepan, combine apricots, orange juice, water, brown sugar and honey. Heat to a boil and reduce temperature to a simmer for 15 minutes. A nice glaze will form.

Remove sweet potatoes from oven and sprinkle with walnuts. Pour the glaze over all. Return to oven for 15 minutes.

Spring Pea-Cheddar Salad

Makes 6 Servings

This dish can be used for several different roles, as a side. Great for lunch, dinner, or a picnic take-a-long. Fresh, tasty, and filled with nutrition, peas are often overlooked as a healthy food. The tomato lacing adds a unique flavor and will be requested by everyone that tries it.

INGREDIENTS:

2 cups fresh or frozen peas, cooked
1 cup cubed Cheddar cheese
2 hardboiled eggs, chopped
¼ cup chopped celery
2 TBSP chopped onion
2 TBSP chopped pimento
1/3 cup homemade mayonnaise
¼ teaspoon hot sauce
1/8 teaspoon pepper
6 tomatoes
Lettuce leaves

INSTRUCTIONS:

In a large mixing bowl, combine peas, cheese, eggs, celery, onion and pimento.

In a smaller bowl, mix together the mayonnaise, hot sauce and pepper.

Pour the sauce over the pea and cheese mixture and stir.

Using a large salad bowl or platter, line with lettuce leaves. Pour the mixture onto the leaves. Cut up the tomatoes into wedges and line up along the outer edges.

Green Bean Casserole Supreme

Makes 8 Servings

The next time someone asks you to bring the green bean casserole, knock them over with this version. A new tradition will be started with fresh green beans, cheese and a touch of lemon. Smooth and delicious, this mellow side compliments any main dish.

INGREDIENTS:

1 pound fresh green beans
1 onion, sliced
1 TBSP fresh parsley
3 TBSP butter
2 TBSP flour substitute
½ teaspoon shredded lemon peel
½ cup milk
1 cup fat-free sour cream
1/8 teaspoon sea salt
¼ teaspoon pepper
½ cup shredded American cheese
¼ cup whole-grain breadcrumbs

INSTRUCTIONS:

Cook the green beans in a large saucepan until tender. Drain and put to the side.

In a large skillet, melt 2 tablespoons of the butter and sauté the onion and parsley. Blend in lemon peel, flour, salt, and pepper. Add milk and stir over medium heat until thickened and bubbly. Add the sour cream and stir until well blended and smooth.

Add the cooked green beans and heat just until bubbly. Remove from heat.

Heat oven to broil.

Spoon the mixture into a 1 ½ quart casserole dish. Spread the shredded cheese on top. Melt the remaining butter and toss with breadcrumbs. Sprinkle these on top of the casserole.

Place in the oven, about 5 inches from the heat and broil for 1-2 minutes, or until the cheese is melted and the crumbs are brown.

Chapter 10: Desserts

Original Angel Food Cake

Makes 12 Servings

Everyone loves an Angel food cake, but the ingredients may not be as rewarding as you may think. Use your new sugar substitute and healthy flour and know that you are eating a healthy dessert. It is not difficult to make your own from scratch with this easy recipe. Served with fresh fruit or drizzled with fruit sauce, this is one dessert that never fails to impress.

INGREDIENTS:

1 ¼ cups healthy flour
¼ teaspoon sea salt
1 teaspoon baking powder
1 ¼ cups sugar substitute
12 egg whites
1 teaspoon cream of tarter
1 teaspoon vanilla flavoring

INSTRUCTIONS:

Warm oven to 350 degrees F.

In a large mixing bowl, beat egg whites and cream of tartar on high speed, using an electric mixer. Add ½ of sugar and continue mixing. Add the remaining sugar and keep mixing until stiff peaks are formed. Add vanilla.

In a separate large bowl, sift the flour, baking powder, and salt. Add slowly into the beaten egg whites, using a rubber spatula to fold into the mix.

Turn the mixture into an ungreased tube pan and bake for 55-60 minutes.

Remove from oven when done and invert onto a pop bottle, or similar device, to allow all sides to cool evenly. When cooled, use a knife to gently loosen the edges and remove to a plate.

Raspberry-Peach Crumble

Makes 8 Servings

This is an old-fashioned favorite that can host a variety of fruits. Rhubarb, pears, apples and blueberries, are other combinations that can replace this raspberry-peach combo. Keep the crumble topping in an air-tight container and have ready for a quick, easy dessert.

INGREDIENTS:

Crumbly Topping

¾ cup healthy flour
¼ cup sugar substitute
¼ packed brown sugar
¾ teaspoon cinnamon
¼ cup chopped walnuts or pecans
6 TBSP melted butter

Filling

¼ cup sugar substitute
2 teaspoons cornstarch
9 fresh peaches, peeled and sliced
1 cup fresh raspberries

INSTRUCTIONS:

Warm oven to 375 degrees F.

In a medium-sized mixing bowl, combine flour, ¼ cup sugar substitute, and cinnamon. Add the melted butter and mix until crumbly. Set aside.

In a small bowl, combine ¼ cup sugar substitute and cornstarch and put to the side.

Using a 3-4 quart baking dish, add sliced peaches. Add cornstarch mixture and toss over peaches. Add raspberries on top and gently fold in to the peaches. Sprinkle the crumbly topping around the peach mixture evenly until the entire top is coated.
Place in the oven and bake for 30 minutes, or until peaches are soft and topping is golden brown. Remove and serve warm.

Classy Carrot Cake

Makes 12-16 Servings

Wow your family and friends with this tantalizing carrot cake that is sweet, healthy and a keeper for anyone who tries it. The original recipe is over 60 years old but they say that classy foods never go out of style. Here is a perfect example.

INGREDIENTS:

3 eggs
1 cup milk
1 TBSP real lemon juice
¾ cup Canola oil
1 ½ cups sugar substitute
2 teaspoons vanilla
2 teaspoons cinnamon
1/8 teaspoon sea salt
2 cups healthy flour
2 teaspoons baking soda
2 cups shredded carrots
1 cup coconut, flaked
1 cup chopped walnuts
½ cup fresh pineapple juice, pulp included
1 cup raisins

INSTRUCTIONS

Heat oven to 350 degrees F.

Use Canola oil spray and lightly put a coat of oil on an 8 x 12 glass baking dish. Sprinkle a coating of flour along the bottom.

Using a medium-sized mixing bowl, combine flour, baking soda, cinnamon and salt. Set aside.

In a large mixing bowl, add eggs, milk, lemon juice, oil, vanilla and sugar. Using an electric beater, mix well. Add the flour mixture and beat until well blended.

Wipe out the medium-sized mixing bowl and add carrots, coconut, walnuts, raisins, and pineapple juice. Blend these ingredients together then transfer to the batter. Use a large wooden spoon or spatula to carefully fold the carrot mixture into the batter. Do not mix.

Pour the batter into the 8 x 12 baking dish and bake for 1 hour. Check with a toothpick through the center for doneness. Remove and cool.

Lemon Bundt Cake with Poppy Seeds

Makes 15 Servings

Enjoy this bundt cake that has an aroma and taste of lemony freshness. It only takes a few roasted poppy seeds to bring out a unique underlying natural flavor. This is a perfect crowd pleaser or to keep on hand as a snack or dessert for the family. No frosting needed for this rich healthy pleasure.

INGREDIENTS:

2 ½ cups healthy flour
1 ½ teaspoons baking powder
½ teaspoon baking soda
1/8 teaspoon sea salt
1 cup milk
3 TBSP freshly squeezed lemon juice
¼ cup toasted poppy seeds
¼ cup Canola oil
1 teaspoon vanilla
2 TBSP grated lemon peel
2 eggs
2 egg whites
1 ¼ cup sugar substitute

INGREDIENTS FOR DRIZZLE TOPPING:

¾ cup confectioner's sugar
3 TBSP freshly squeezed lemon juice
1 TBSP water

INSTRUCTIONS:

Warm oven to 350 degrees F.

Spray the interior of a bundt pan with Canola spray and dust lightly with flour.

In a large mixing bowl, combine flour, poppy seeds, baking powder, baking soda, and sea salt. Mix together.

In a 2-cup measuring cup, add milk, lemon juice, and lemon peel.
In a separate large mixing bowl, add eggs, egg whites, and sugar. Beat with an electric mixer on high speed until thickened, about 5 minutes.

Fold 1/3 of the flour mixture into the egg mixture and blend well with a rubber spatula or large wooden spoon. Add 1/3 of the milk mixture and blend lightly. Repeat this process until all the ingredients have been added and blended.

Spoon all contents into the bundt pan and smooth evenly. Place in oven and bake for 35-40 minutes. Test with a toothpick to insure doneness. Remove from oven and cool for about 5 minutes before inverting onto a wire rack.

To make the glaze, combine the confectioner's sugar with the lemon juice and water in a small mixing bowl and blend until smooth. Turn the cake right side up onto a serving platter. Poke holes along the top of the cake, then spread the glaze along the top with a pastry brush. Top it off with a dusting of sifted confectioner's sugar.

Peanut Butter Cookies-Hold the Flour

Makes 18 Servings

Who says you need flour to bake up a batch of warm and delicious cookies? This recipe contains no flour and the flavor of peanut butter is, oh so rich. 4 main ingredients and 30 minutes of baking is all that is required to whip up a dessert that will be gone in seconds.

INGREDIENTS:

1 cup natural peanut butter
1 egg
1 cup sugar substitute
1 teaspoon vanilla
sea salt
honey

INSTRUCTIONS:

Position 1 oven rack in upper 1/3 of oven and place a second rack in the lower 1/3 part of the oven. Heat oven to 350 degrees F.

In a medium-sized mixing bowl, combine peanut butter,

egg, sugar substitute, and vanilla. Stir until all is well combined.

Drop by a tablespoon onto an ungreased cookie sheet, keeping 1 inch apart from each other. Flatten with a fork in a crisscross design and sprinkle with sea salt.

Bake in oven for 5 minutes on upper rack. Move to lower rack for another 5 minutes. Continue baking until golden brown along the edges. Remove and transfer to waxed paper. Drizzle with a little warmed honey.

Perfect Strawberry Parfait

Makes 4 Servings

Finish your dinner with this sweet and light dessert that is always a pleaser. Fresh strawberries, amaretto cookie pieces, and ricotta cheese, will tempt your taste buds, without adding on a heavy feeling of too many rich carbohydrates.

INGREDIENTS:

4 cups fresh sliced strawberries
1 cup fat-free ricotta cheese
4 ounces softened low-fat cream cheese
½ cup sugar substitute
8 amaretto cookies, crushed
1 teaspoon vanilla
4 TBSP almond slivers

INSTRUCTIONS:

Using a blender, puree 2 cups strawberries and ¼ cup sugar substitute. Remove to a bowl and set aside.

In a medium-sized bowl, mix the ricotta cheese, cream cheese, ¼ cup sugar substitute, and vanilla. Add a little water if mixture is too thick.

Use 4 parfait glasses and begin assembling the parfaits by putting 2 tablespoons crushed cookies in the bottom of each glass. Add 2 tablespoons strawberry puree, ¼ cup sliced strawberries, then cream cheese mixture. Repeat until the glasses are filled. Top with 1 tablespoon almond slivers.

Chapter 11: Snacks

Caribbean Fruitsicles

Makes 6 Servings

If you love sherbet, you will be amazed with these homemade fruity popsicles that really hit the spot. You will also find that coconut juice is one of the most thirst quenching drinks that can be found. If you don't have iced-pop makers, use any type of heavy plastic container or ice cube trays. This is a great treat for kids and adults, alike.

INGREDIENTS:

1 cup fresh coconut water
2 ripened bananas
1 pitted date
3 strawberries, cut in quarters
6 blueberries, cut in half

INSTRUCTIONS:

Combine coconut water, bananas and date in a blender.

Blend on high. If the bananas begin to make the liquid sticky, add a little more coconut water. Blend until milky and smooth. Pour into containers and drop in chunks of strawberries and blueberries and freeze.

Snackin' Cranberry Granola

Makes 6 Servings

Whip up a batch of this finger snack food and keep in an air-tight container on the counter. There will be no more rummaging through cabinets and the refrigerator as your after school gang makes a bee-line for this sweet and crunchy snack. It might be a good idea to make plenty of back-up granola and store off-site.

INGREDIENTS:

2 cups natural rolled oats
1 cup sliced almonds
½ cup dried cranberries
1 teaspoon cinnamon
1/8 teaspoon sea salt
4 TBSP butter
¼ cup quality honey
¼ cup brown sugar
1 teaspoon vanilla

INSTRUCTIONS:

Heat oven to 400 degrees F.

Use aluminum foil and place over a cookie sheet. Spray lightly with Canola oil.

In a large mixing bowl, add rolled oats, almonds, cranberries, and cinnamon. Mix together.

Use a saucepan on the stove and add sugar, butter and honey. Melt on low heat and increase to medium to get the mixture to a boil. Add vanilla and remove from heat and stir.

Pour the honey mixture over the oats and toss with a large wooden spoon or rubber spatula. Turn all onto the prepared cookie sheet and spread out evenly. Bake for 20-25 minutes. Check to see if oats have turned a golden brown. If so, remove from oven and let cool.

Break up the granola into bite-sized pieces and place in an air-tight container.

Vanilla Lovers Granola

Makes 16 Servings

Nothing says home like the fresh scent of vanilla that drifts throughout a kitchen. This recipe will attract visitors like bees to honey with a soothing aroma, and even better taste. Open the air-tight container about 30 minutes before the crowd comes in and watch as they search for the delightful snack.

INGREDIENTS:

4 cups natural rolled oats
1 cup sliced almonds
½ cup brown sugar substitute
1/8 teaspoon sea salt
1/8 teaspoon cinnamon
1/3 cup canola oil
¼ cup quality honey
2 tablespoons sugar substitute
4 teaspoons vanilla

INSTRUCTIONS:

Place oven rack in center of oven and heat to 300 degrees F. Spray large baking sheet with canola oil.

In a large mixing bowl, add rolled oats, almonds, brown sugar substitute, sea salt and cinnamon. Toss well.

Using a small saucepan, add oil, honey and sugar. Heat to boiling and remove. Add vanilla and stir. Allow to cool slightly and pour over the oat mixture.

Using a large wood spoon or your hands, toss the ingredients until all is well coated.

Transfer the contents to the greased baking pan and smooth out over the surface as evenly as possible.

Bake for about 30 minutes, or until rolled oats are a golden brown. Remove from oven and allow to cool. Break up into clusters and place in an air-tight container.

Bugs on a Log

Makes 4 Servings

This makeover of Ants on a Log, never loses its wit. By using plain old celery and dressing up a bit, the kids will have fun and stay away from the chips and candy. This treat can also be a snack during a day at work or just to have something healthy to munch on. Sometimes, you just have to put something in your mouth, so make it the best it can be.

INGREDIENTS:

4 strips of celery from a stalk
4 TBSP almond or peanut butter
½ cup raisins
¼ cup almonds

INSTRUCTIONS:

Wash and air dry the celery strips then cut in half lengthwise. Next, cut the pieces in thirds. Line up and spread the almond or peanut butter on each stick.

Use your choice of raisins or almonds and place 2 or 3 in the butter of each.

Apple-Cinnamon Chips

Makes 2 Servings

Potato chips can be addictive but not for long when you find a treat that is crunchy and not as greasy. Make these apple-cinnamon chips instead of grabbing a bag of processed chips and get the crunch while saving your health. Light and crispy, you will soon have a new addiction to crave.

INGREDIENTS:

4 apples
1 ½ teaspoons cinnamon
¼ teaspoon allspice
½ teaspoon nutmeg
pinch of sea salt
2 TBSP sugar substitute

INSTRUCTIONS:

Warm oven to 200 degrees F. Use parchment paper and place over a cookie sheet.

Leaving the skin on, chop the ends off of each apple. You are going to slice your apples as thin as possible, about 1/8 inch or thinner. Don't worry about removing the seeds. They will fall out as you slice.

Use a small bowl and combine the cinnamon, allspice, nutmeg, salt and sugar substitute. Coat each slice in the mixture, on both sides. Shake off any excess.

Arrange on the cookie sheet and parchment paper in a single layer. Bake for 30 minutes. Remove from oven and carefully turn each apple slice over. Bake for an additional 10-15 minutes. The apple slices may remain flat but have a dried appearance. This is the time the remove from the oven. After cooling for a few minutes, watch as the ends begin to curl. Eat plain or dip in cottage cheese, yogurt or a little honey.

Fruit-Nutty Trail Mix

Makes 6 Servings

Trail Mix that you buy in a store may seem like a healthy snack until you look at the ingredients and additives. This product is made to last a long time on your grocer's shelves and in order to do that, the contents need to be preserved. Save your money and make your own natural trail mix that is guaranteed to be fresh and natural.

INGREDIENTS:

¼ cup raw cashews
¼ cup raw almonds
¼ cup walnut halves
¼ cup dried apricots
¼ cup dried cranberries
¼ cup dried bananas
¼ cup raisins
sea salt

INSTRUCTIONS:

Heat oven to 350 degrees F.

Place the cashews, almonds and walnuts in a medium-sized bowl and add a pinch of sea salt. Stir around then pour onto a baking sheet. Separate as much as possible and bake for 7 minutes. Remove and stir. Return to oven for an additional 5 minutes. Remove from oven and allow to cool.

Using the same bowl as the nuts were in, add the apricots, cranberries, bananas, and raisins. Pour the cooled nuts on top. Mix together and store in an air-tight container.

Get creative with your trail mix by substituting different nuts, dried fruits or adding coconut or dark chocolate. If you have a favorite type at the store, make a list of the contents and create your own. Homemade trail mix will last for 4 days and is healthier, and better tasting that store-bought.

Chapter 12: Beverages

Green Tea/Mango Surprise

Makes 3 Servings

Make a tropical beverage by using green tea as a base. Mango nectar is known for having a wide variety of important minerals and vitamins. When these two healthy forces meet, you know that you have a winner. Keep a sprig of mint handy for garnish.

INGREDIENTS:

1 cup brewed green tea (use 2 bags)
2 cups mango nectar
1 mango, cut into six slices
2 cups ice cubes

INSTRUCTIONS:

Allow the brewed green tea to cool. Place the tea, nectar and ice cubes in a blender. Blend until smooth. Pour into 3 glasses and add a couple mango sections to each glass.

Homemade Honey Lemonade

Makes 6 Servings

The trick behind any great-tasting homemade lemonade is in steeping the pulp of the lemons first. Also, soften up your lemons before squeezing by placing in the microwave for 30 seconds. This will help loosen the juice from the skin. Once you have this method down pat, there will always be a pitcher of fresh lemonade in the frig for thirsty little mouths.

INGREDIENTS:

1 cup fresh squeezed lemon juice (4-5 lemons)
½ cup quality honey
6 cups chilled water

INSTRUCTIONS:

Use a saucepan and add the lemon juice and honey together. Heat until blended then refrigerate. This can be made a couple hours ahead of time.

In a large pitcher, combine the lemon and honey mixture to the chilled water and mix well.

Tip – Replace honey with 1 ½ cups sugar substitute if looking to make the old fashioned lemonade version.

Peachy Spritzer

Makes 6 Servings

How come all of the really great tasting drinks are laced with alcohol and called cocktails? Guess what, you can turn those recipes into healthy, refreshing drinks, without the pain tomorrow morning. Here is an example of a vitamin-enriched drink that is sure to please-hold the vodka, please.

INGREDIENTS:

1 quart chilled homemade lemonade
2 cups chilled peach nectar
1 liter chilled sparkling white grape juice
2 cups fresh raspberries
2 fresh peaches, sliced thick

INSTRUCTIONS:

Using a tall pitcher, mix the lemonade and nectar. Add the grape juice and stir. Add raspberries on top.

Pour into glasses filled with crushed ice and add a peach slice on the rim.

Famous Fruity Smoothie

Makes 3 Servings

This amazing smoothie can also be classified as a snack or dessert because it takes care of hunger and is rich and sweet. But unlike unhealthy drinks or foods that fill you with empty calories, this one is packed full of nutrients and energy-enhancing fruits.

INGREDIENTS:

1 ripe, sliced banana
1 cup fresh squeezed orange juice
1 cup peeled, sliced peaches
1 cup halved strawberries
1 TBSP honey

INSTRUCTIONS:

Combine all ingredients in a blender and blend until smooth. Pour into glasses with shaved ice.

Chocolate Covered Banana Milkshake

Makes 1 Serving

This recipe would certainly make Elvis a happy man. Bananas, peanut butter and chocolate, are a heavenly combination for taking the edge off of your desire to indulge. But believe it or not, all of these ingredients are healthy and non-fattening. So treat yourself and never feel bad.

INGREDIENTS:

1 banana
2 TBSP cacao powder
2 TBSP peanut or almond butter
2 TBSP coconut
1/3 cup water

INSTRUCTIONS:

Place all ingredients in a blender and mix until smooth. Adjust the water content to your liking. You can omit the coconut, add 2 TBSP rolled oats, or a pinch of cinnamon to your personal taste and consistency.

Honeydew Delight

Makes 2 Servings

Melon is a perfect form of nutrition in the summer months. Try this smoothie recipe and enjoy sipping the flavors while enjoying the weather. Cucumbers and oranges add a zing to the mild flavor of honeydew.

INGREDIENTS:

2 cups fresh honeydew, cubed and frozen
1 peeled orange
1 cup sliced cucumber
½ cup Greek yogurt
1 TBSP fresh lemon juice
10 ice cubes

INSTRUCTIONS:

Place all ingredients in a blender and mix until smooth.

Caribbean Cooler

Makes 1 Serving

Picture the beautiful waves of the Caribbean while you sit by the pool and close your eyes. The natural flavors of coconut, pineapple and sweet oranges will almost make you feel the soothing, healing waters, as you enjoy this tropical cooler.

INGREDIENTS:

¼ cup fresh pineapple juice
¼ cup fresh orange juice
1 banana
1 TBSP coconut milk
¼ teaspoon fresh ginger root
3 ice cubes

INSTRUCTIONS:

In a blender, add all ingredients and blend until smooth and creamy.

Clean Eating Conclusion

Many of the recipes that you have read in this book, do not appear to be much different than the foods you are currently eating. The main difference is in the homemade goodness that puts you in charge of what your body wants and needs.

Packaged foods, canned goods, refined sugar and bleached flour, are a few of the items that are scarce in these great-tasting meals and drinks. By eliminating chemicals, dyes and additives that are harmful to your system, you will be able to better enjoy the taste, balance your hormones, and lose that stubborn weight. While the Clean Diet is not designed to shed fat overnight, your body will soon return to a natural lean exterior.

Less tiredness, more energy and a renewed zest for life is the outcome that we hope to introduce to you through learning the truth about the foods you eat. The choice is yours, but most people would rather have a healthy body, a better attitude and a future to look forward to.

It may take some practice to find the right blend of

flours that create the flavor you are looking for, but once it is found, you will never use regular white flour again. The same holds true for refined sugar. The choices are wide, as are the different tastes, but you will find them all, very appealing.

Eating clean does not involve counting calories, balancing carbs or looking for fat-free products. What it does provide, is a chance to return your body to its original condition, before the introduction of preservatives. If this idea seems a little old-fashioned to you, that's because it is, in our country. All around the world, cultures are enjoying long lives, little disease and even, better looking skin. Life should not be a race to get to the next destination, but a time to enjoy all the pleasures along the way. One of those delights can be from enjoying food once again, with the Clean Diet.

Section 2: Belly Fat Diet

Even if you have lost weight and you have toned up your body, you may still be dealing with stubborn belly fat. Belly fat is difficult to lose. You may be working out and trying to eat right, but it may seem that your belly just refuses to get flatter. If this is a problem you are dealing with, the belly fat diet may be the right diet for your needs. This diet is specifically designed to help you lose belly fat now. The foods included in the diet help target belly fat, helping you finally get rid of that belly.

This book is packed with all the information you need to successfully follow the belly fat diet and lose belly fat now. You will find helpful information on the diet, the benefits of following this diet and more. As you get started on the diet, you can enjoy using some of the helpful tips provided to ensure you are successful when you begin using this diet. The best part of this book is the many powerful recipes that will help support your belly melt diet. You will not have to start searching for recipes that go with your new diet.

Recipes are included for every meal. Great breakfast recipes will help you start out your day the right way. Tasty lunch recipes will keep you fueled up during the day and help you avoid cravings. The dinner recipes included will help you enjoy tasty meals that even your family will enjoy and many of them are ready in only a short amount of time, allowing you to add healthy eating to your busy life. You may be surprised to find dessert and snack recipes as well. Enjoy a delicious dessert or snack without sabotaging your belly fat diet.

You can finally get rid of that belly you have had for so long. Use these tips and the delicious recipes and included and you will quickly be on your way to a flatter belly.

Chapter 1: What is the Belly Fat Diet?

What is the belly fat diet? Maybe you have heard about this diet but you are not quite sure what it is and how it works. Basically, the belly fat diet is a special diet that is designed to help you take off inches of belly fat. You will lose weight while you are on this diet. However, the important part to note is that you will be taking off belly fat, not just losing a few pounds. While every individual is difference, most people end up losing 12-15 pounds within a month when they follow this diet. Several inches of belly fat are usually lost as well. The great thing about the diet is that you will not have to do hundreds of crunches to enjoy a flatter belly.

The Secret Behind the Diet

There is one big secret behind the diet – MUFAs. What are MUFAs? They are monounsaturated fatty acids. These fatty acids work to eliminate belly fat and they also make you feel full. Not only will you melt away belly fat when adding MUFAs to your diet, but these fatty acids will keep you feeling satisfied, which can help keep you from overeating as well. MUFAs are plant based fats and they can be found in foods like olive oil, chocolate, seeds, avocados and nuts. To get the best results while on this diet, you should strive to get a serving of MUFAs with every meal that you eat.

Even though MUFAs are fatty acids, these are healthy fats. They will not clog up your arteries. Instead, they actually help to improve your health. Along with the emphasis on MUFAs, which is the big secret behind this diet, the diet also emphasizes eating key foods like whole grains, fish, veggies, fruits, legumes and olive oil. In fact, this diet includes foods that are often found within the Mediterranean approach to eating.

How the Diet Works

Now that you know the secret behind the diet, you may be wondering how the diet works. The diet focuses on eating about 1600 calories a day and also involves eating a serving of MUFAs with each meal that you eat. Of course, keep in mind that you can tailor the number of calories you take in to your gender, activity level and your age. The diet includes avoiding processed, high fat foods. While protein is an important part of each meal, the focus is on vegetables and fruits with each meal.

The great thing about this diet is that most people find it very easy to follow. While you will have to restrict your diet to some extent, you still are able to enjoy wonderful meals that include delicious dishes. Many of the recipes included with this diet are easy to prepare, which makes this diet easy to follow, even for individuals that are very busy. You will not have to worry about skimping on taste either. Enjoy chocolate dishes, veggie pizzas and other great recipes that are sure to keep your taste buds happy.

Chapter 2: Benefits of the Belly Fat Diet

Belly fat, while it can be unsightly, can actually have serious long term health consequences. While going on the belly fat diet can help you lose your belly and feel better about the way you look, the main benefits of losing belly fat are health benefits. Unfortunately, while belly fat can be so dangerous, it is also extremely difficult to lose. Going on the belly fat diet can help blast away that belly fat. While you may already be excited about trying this diet, here are a few of the top benefits you can enjoy with this diet, which may excite you even more.

Benefit #1 – Reduce the Risk of Diabetes and Heart Disease

One of the best benefits of going on the belly fat diet is that it can help to reduce your risk of diabetes and heart disease. Excess belly fat can drastically increase your risk of developing diseases like diabetes and heart disease. In fact, excess belly fat can be almost as dangerous as smoking when it comes to increasing your risk of diseases like heart disease. The great news is that you can eliminate belly fat as a major risk factor for diabetes and heart disease. By following the belly fat diet, you can reduce your belly fat and begin reducing your risk of dealing with diabetes or heart disease in the future. In fact, your overall health will be improved as you melt that belly fat away.

Benefit #2 – Keep Testosterone Levels Normal

Studies show that having too much belly fat may lead to a reduction in testosterone within the body. This is especially troublesome for men, although women have testosterone as well. Low testosterone in men often causes impotence and lack of libido. The good news is that losing that belly fat can help keep testosterone at normal levels. Eliminating belly fat naturally begins to bring up testosterone levels. Adding exercise to the belly fat diet will boost levels of testosterone even more.

Benefit #3 – Enjoy Better Sleep at Night

Newer research that was done by Johns Hopkins shows that those who have more belly fat may not sleep as well as those with little belly fat. Losing belly fat may actually improve sleep quality. The study showed that those who reduced abdominal fat actually improved their sleep quality assessment test scores. This is important, since lack of sleep can cause a range of different health problems, including heart disease, depression and more. Simply losing some belly fat may be enough to help you sleep better, avoiding chronic lack of sleep.

Benefit #4 – Feel Better About Yourself

Last, the belly fat diet can help you blast away that troublesome belly fat, which has the benefit of helping you feel better about yourself. You may have a negative self-image of yourself while you still have belly fat. Losing the belly fat can help you improve your self-image, becoming happier with the way you look and feel. You may also enjoy feeling satisfied and triumphant when you succeed at improving your body and your health with the belly fat diet.

Chapter 3: Essential Tips for Success on the Belly Melt Diet

As you begin your belly fat diet, you want to ensure that you are successful. It can be easy to let a busy life get you off track when you are on a diet or to fall back into old habits that sabotage your efforts. To help you make the most of this diet, we have put together some great diet tips that will boost your belly melting efforts. You will also find a closer look at some of the top belly fat burning foods that you can work to add to this diet on a regular basis. With this information to guide you, you will have no problem making this diet successful.

Helpful Diet Tips to Follow

While the belly fat diet focuses on reducing calories, adding MUFAs and eating wholesome foods, there are some other tips you can follow to make the most of this diet. To help you get better results as you work to lose that belly fat, here are some helpful diet tips you definitely want to follow as you go on the belly fat diet.

- **Tip #1 – Avoid Drinking Your Calories** – On the belly fat diet, you should be taking in about 1600 calories each day. One of your best tips for success is to avoid drinking your calories. You may be surprised to find that many tasty drinks like shakes, juices and some coffee beverages can have hundreds of calories in a single drink. This quickly takes a big bite out of the calories you are supposed to have each day. Another big problem is that most of the calories in these drinks come from sugar, which can actually make your body store more belly fat instead of losing it. Instead of drinking your calories, focus on drinking plenty of water. You can also drink black coffee and certain teas without adding calories to your diet. Making this one simple change to your diet as you take on the belly fat diet can make a huge difference and help you lose that belly fat faster.

- **Tip #2 – Stay Away From Anything Processed and Refined** – Another helpful diet tip to follow while you are on the belly melt diet is to stay away from anything that is processed and refined. Processed foods usually have their nutrients stripped away when they are refined. They may also include many additives and sugar. That added sugar can make you feel hungrier, lead to more fat storage and can increase the production of insulin within your body. Processed, refined foods will sabotage your belly fat diet. Stay away from them and you are sure to enjoy better results.

- **Tip #3 – Don't Be Afraid to Cheat Once a Week** – It can be difficult to stick to a new diet all the time, especially if you are craving a specific food that you cannot have on your new diet. To make sure you stick with this belly fat diet, do not be afraid to cheat once a week. On one day, allow yourself to have one dessert that you have been craving or let yourself eat one cheeseburger or a slice of pizza. Knowing that you can cheat once a week can help you stick to your diet during the rest of the week. Feeling deprived can make you fail at your diet. Instead of feeling deprived, remind yourself that once each week you can enjoy cheating for a meal. It will go a long way towards helping you stick with the belly fat diet as you blast that fat away for good.

Top Belly Fat Burning Foods

While MUFAs are one of the big secrets to this belly fat diet, there are many other great belly fat burning foods that you can add to your diet to help you melt that belly fat. Here is a look at some of the top belly fat burning foods you should be eating and information on why they help you eliminate belly fat.

- **Fruits Rich in Fiber** – It is important to have plenty of fruits in your diet, especially those that are rich in fiber. They help make sure you get all the vitamins and minerals that your body needs. Berries are particularly important, since they are high in antioxidants and will help blast away belly fat. Some of the other great fruits that you should eat while on this diet include papayas, oranges, watermelon, peaches, cantaloupes, apples and apricots. Just make sure you eat fruits raw instead of drinking fruit juices.

- **Fiber Rich Veggies** – Veggies are an important part of your belly fat diet and they help make sure your body is burning off fat effectively. Some of the best vegies include leafy greens like cabbage, kale, lettuces and spinach. Other great veggies include cucumbers, broccoli, tomatoes and zucchini. Veggies can be eaten in salads, added to soups, stir fried, steamed or added to other dishes. The great thing about fiber rich veggies is that they fill you up and help to fight off cravings, which helps make it easier to lose belly fat.

- **Eggs** – Eggs are a powerful belly fat burning food to eat while following the belly fat diet. They have important vitamins that help your body burn fat. Eggs also have a lot of protein, which keeps you feeling full as well. Poach eggs, scramble them or even eat them hard boiled. They make a great breakfast that will fuel you for your day and help boost your belly melting efforts.

- **Green Tea** – Adding green tea to your belly fat diet is a great idea for several reasons. First, it works by flushing toxins out of your body naturally, eliminating water retention and bloating. It also has compounds that are known to help with weight loss, giving your metabolism a boost. Add a bit of lemon juice and honey to the tea for a very low calorie drink that will help burn fat.

- **Beans** – Different types of beans are a great addition to your belly fat diet as well. Beans are very high in protein, which can help to blast away stomach fat. Some great beans to try include Edamame, garbanzo beans, chick peas, kidney beans and black beans. Of course, when you add beans to your diet, avoid consuming them in large amounts. Too many beans can lead to bloating and gas, which will make your belly feel bigger.

These are just a few of the excellent foods that should be included in your belly fat diet. Along with the addition of MUFAs, they can help to blast away belly fat, helping you to enjoy success as you take on this new diet plan.

Chapter 4: Belly Melting Breakfast Recipes

Breakfast is the most important meal of your day, especially when you are trying to lose belly fat. On the belly fat diet, you need to make sure you get a good breakfast in your stomach to keep you feeling full until lunch. These recipes are packed with protein, fiber and healthy fats, helping you feel satisfied while ensuring you enjoy what you're eating.

Banana Walnut Breakfast Muffin Recipe

These delicious muffins make any breakfast special, including all the flavors you'd expect to find in a banana split. The great thing about these muffins is that they are perfect for your belly fat diet too. Breakfast will almost feel like dessert when you make these muffins for breakfast. In fact, you may want to make a few extras and freeze them to enjoy at a later date.

What You'll Need:

¾ cup of mini chocolate chips, semisweet
1 ½ cups of walnuts, chopped
¼ cup of canola oil
1 banana, very ripe and mashed
½ cup of dark brown sugar, packed
1 ½ cups of all-purpose flour
1 large egg
¼ cup of Greek yogurt, plain
½ teaspoon of ground cinnamon
¼ cup of skim milk
1 teaspoon of vanilla
1 tablespoon of baking powder
½ teaspoon of salt

How to Make It:

Start by preheating the oven to 375F. Add muffin papers to a muffin pan or use cooking spray to prepare a 12 cup muffin pan.

Add a half cup of walnuts to a food processor, processing until you have a very find powder. Next, place the freshly ground walnuts, baking powder, salt, flour, cinnamon, and chocolate chips in a large mixing bowl. Mix and combine thoroughly.

In a medium sized mixing bowl, combine the milk, vanilla, oil, egg, brown sugar, banana and yogurt. Stir until the mixture becomes smooth. Combine the flour and banana mixtures together, combining well. Last, stir the last cup of chopped walnuts into the batter. The batter should be quite thick.

Fill each muffin cup with the batter until about ¾ of the way full. Place muffins in the oven, allowing to bake for about 15 minutes. Check muffins for doneness. If the tops lightly spring back when you touch them, they are done. Remove muffins from the oven. Allow to sit for a few minutes. Then, remove each muffin from the muffin tin, placing them on a rack to cool. Makes 12 muffins.

Tomato Pesto Eggs Florentine Breakfast Recipe

A recipe from Prevention.com inspires this tasty recipe. It is easy to make, even for those who have never poached eggs in the past. While this recipe is wonderful for any breakfast, it makes a wonderful dish to serve guests for a nice brunch. It offers a nice mixture of protein, carbs and veggies, getting you ready for your shape. The bit of vinegar added to the recipe helps the egg whites to keep their shape while cooking.

What You'll Need:

1/3 cup of Greek yogurt, fat free
4 large eggs
1 teaspoon of olive oil
1 teaspoon of vinegar
1 9-oz package of baby spinach, prewashed
2 English muffins, whole grain, split and then toasted
¼ cup of sun-dried tomato pesto
Ground black pepper, freshly ground
Pinch of salt

How to Make It:

In a large skillet, heat up the olive oil on medium heat. One oil is hot, add spinach to the pan, cooking it just until it wilts. In a small bowl, combine the sun-dried tomato pesto and the yogurt. Then, stir a ¼ cup of the mixture into the spinach, immediate removing the spinach from the heat. Cover the skillet, keeping the spinach warm.

Meanwhile, add about 1 inch of water to a medium saucepan, heating it up on medium heat until it begins to boil. Once it starts boiling, add the salt and vinegar, turning the heat down to low. Break an egg into a small cup, then gently place the egg in the hot water. Do the same thing with each egg. Cover the pan, allowing the water to simmer. Cooking for about 3-5 minutes, shaking from a couple times. Yolks should start thickening and whites should be set when the eggs are done.

One four warmed plates, place half of an English muffin. Place about ¼ of the spinach mixture over the muffin. With a slotted spoon, remove poached eggs, draining them and placing on top of the spinach. Add a tablespoon of the poaching water to the leftover yogurt mixture, stirring it until smooth. Spread the yogurt mixture over eggs. Top with a bit of freshly ground pepper and serve right away. Makes four servings.

Pumpkin Pie Flavored Oatmeal Breakfast Recipe

This is a delicious belly fat buster that tastes amazing. You get the wonderful taste of pumpkin pie while blasting away belly fat. You'll also find that this oatmeal recipe is very filling, helping you avoid cravings throughout your day. Serve up this oatmeal with about a cup of skim milk. This only makes a single serving, so you may want to double or quadruple the recipe if you need to make more.

What You'll Need:

1/3 cup of quick cooking oats
1 teaspoons of brown sugar
1 cup of water
¼ cup of canned pure pumpkin (not pumpkin pie filling)
Pinch of ground cloves
Pinch of nutmeg
Pinch of salt
¼ teaspoon of ground cinnamon
2 tablespoons of pecans, chopped and toasted

How to Make It:

Heat up the water in a medium saucepan. Heat until water is boiling. After water comes to a boil, add the quick oats and the salt to the pan. Allow to cook for about 90 seconds. In a small bowl, combine the pumpkin, brown sugar, cloves, nutmeg, cinnamon and pecans. Reduce the heat of the oatmeal, once on low, stir the pumpkin pecan mixture into the oatmeal. Serve with skim milk. Makes a single serving.

Delicious French Toast with Chocolate Breakfast Recipe

If you have a bit of extra time on the weekend, this recipe is sure to be a hit with the family while going along with your belly fat diet. The great thing about this wonderful French toast recipe is that it offers plenty of fiber and protein for breakfast, which helps to keep you feeling full. Add fruit on the side for a well-rounded breakfast that you're sure to enjoy. After all, it's always nice to start the day with a bit of chocolate.

What You'll Need:

3 ounces of low fat cream cheese, softened
6 ounces of Italian bread, cut into 8 slices about a half inch thick
2 large egg whites
2 large eggs
4 ounces of semi-sweet chocolate, chopped finely
1 tablespoon of margarine, trans fat free
1 tablespoon of sugar
1 teaspoon of vanilla
1 teaspoon of orange zest, freshly grated
2 cups of fresh strawberries, sliced

How to Make It:

In a little bowl, combine the cream cheese and the chocolate together. In another bowl, combine the orange zest, sugar and strawberry slices.

On four slices of the Italian bread, spread a quarter of the cream cheese and chocolate mixture. Top each slice with another slice of bread, pressing slices together lightly.

In a medium sized bowl, combine the vanilla, egg whites and eggs. Whip lightly. Dip each side of the bread into the egg mixture, then setting the sandwich on a platter.

Place margarine in a large skillet, heating it on medium heat. When margarine is completely melted, place sandwiches into the skillet, cooking for about four minutes on each side. French toast should be cooked through and golden brown. Divide the fresh toast among four plates, topping the fresh toast with the strawberry mixture. Serve while hot. Makes four servings.

Belly Melt Huevos Racheros Breakfast Recipe

When you try this delicious breakfast recipe, you'll be surprised at all the flavor. It includes plenty of veggies and wonderful herbs add tons of flavor. The eggs give you plenty of protein, while you get your monounsaturated fats from the avocado that is included. If you like a little more kick when you eat your eggs, try adding just a bit of hot pepper sauce to the eggs when you eat them.

What You'll Need:

4 scallions, thinly sliced
1 teaspoon of ground cumin
2 cloves of garlic, minced
4 tablespoons of salsa
1 cup of avocado, sliced
½ cup of chicken broth, reduced-sodium
1 can of pink beans, no salt added, drained and rinsed
1 red bell pepper, sliced into thin strips
4 tablespoons of Greek yogurt, fat free
4 eggs
8 six-inch corn tortillas, toasted

How to Make It:

Begin heating a 10-inch skillet on medium heat. Place cumin in the pan, allowing to cook until it becomes fragrant. Only cook for about 30 seconds, stirring from time to time. Place the garlic, bell pepper, beans, broth and scallions in the skillet with the cumin. Bring the mixture to a boil, then reduce heat, allowing the mixture to simmer. Simmer for about eight minutes, ensuring that the vegetables become very tender and most of the chicken broth evaporates. Use a spoon to smash up the beans, making a thick, lumpy mixture.

With the back of a wooden spoon, make four different indentations in the mixture. Break an egg into a cup, pouring carefully into one of the indentations. Do the same thing with the rest of the eggs. Cover the skillet and allow eggs to cook for 8-10 minutes, ensuring that eggs are done to your taste.

Separate the mixture into four equal parts, ensuring each part has one egg. Place on four plates. Place slices of avocado around the beans. Use the salsa and yogurt to top the dish. Serve up with the toasted tortillas while hot. Makes four servings.

Belly Filling Parfait with Granola Breakfast Recipe

Not only is this parfait a delicious treat, but it is good for you to. You can make it in no time, which makes it great for busy mornings. It also looks elegant, which means you can serve this healthy breakfast up to guests and they'll never know how healthy it really is for them.

What You'll Need:

1 cup of raspberries
1 ½ cups of Granola
1 large banana, sliced
1 small 5.3 ounce container of Greek yogurt, fat free

How to Make It:

Place a small amount of granola in the bottom of a tall glass or parfait cup. Top with granola. Add fruit on top of granola. Repeat layers until the glass is full. Do the same thing in the second glass. Makes two servings, but it's easy to double the recipe to make more.

Decadent Walnut Banana Pancakes Breakfast Recipe

These pancakes are sensational and they'll help you work on gaining a flat belly too. You get a nice combination of crunchy and sweet with the walnuts and honey included in the recipe. The walnuts also add healthy, belly blasting fats to the recipe as well. This recipe includes plenty of fiber too, which means you'll stay feeling full longer. Serve with berries on the side for the perfect breakfast.

What You'll Need:

¼ cup of water
1 tablespoon of canola oil
½ cup of fresh raspberries
1 1/3 pancake mix, trans fat free
1 egg
1 teaspoon of vanilla
1 cup of buttermilk, low fat
¼ teaspoon of ground cinnamon
1 large banana, cut into very thin slices

1/3 cup of honey
1 tablespoon of water
½ cup of chopped walnuts

How to Make It:

In a large mixing bowl, combine the cinnamon and pancake mix. In a smaller bowl, combine the vanilla, egg, oil, buttermilk and water. Whisk the wet ingredients into the dry ingredients, stirring well until you have a smooth mixture. Fold the slices of banana into the pancake batter, setting to the side.

In a small bowl, combine the water, honey and walnuts.

Take a large nonstick skillet, coating it well with cooking spray. Place on medium heat and warm. Once the skillet is hot, begin adding batter by the ¼ cupful, cooking in batches. Pancakes should cook for about 2 minutes on each side, or until they become browned lightly.

Serve up pancakes, dividing among four separate plates. While hot, top with the walnut and honey mixture. Serve the raspberries on the side. Makes four servings.

Pecan and Cranberry Scones Breakfast Recipe

When you want a nice treat for breakfast, these scones are the perfect option. You can easily make a nice batch of the scones at the beginning of the week, storing them in the freezer so you can enjoy them all week. In fact, they are great if you need to grab your breakfast when you're headed out the door. The pecans add the monounsaturated fat to the recipe, helping it blast away your belly fat while enjoying a delicious breakfast.

What You'll Need:

1 ¼ cup of vanilla yogurt, low fat
1 cup of chopped pecans
2/3 cup of sweetened, dried cranberries
2 tablespoons of canola oil
2 cups of whole wheat pastry flour
½ teaspoon of baking soda
1 teaspoon of orange zest, freshly grated
½ teaspoon of salt
2 teaspoons of baking powder

How to Make It:

Preheat oven to 400F.

Coat a 9-inch round baking dish with some nonstick cooking spray.

In a large mixing bowl, mix together the baking powder, salt, baking soda, pecans and flour. In a smaller bowl, combine the orange zest, oil and yogurt. In the middle of the flour mixture, create a well, pouring the yogurt mixture into the well, as well as the cranberries. Stir the mixture until ingredients are blended.

Press the batter into the pan that has been prepared with cooking spray. Use a knife to score the dough, making eight triangles. Bake the scones for about 20-25 minutes. To check for doneness, insert a toothpick into the center. It should come out clean if the scones are done. Makes eight servings.

Nut and Fruit Oatmeal Breakfast Recipe

You probably already know how great oatmeal is for your heart. However, you may be unaware of how great it is for flattening your belly. This oatmeal recipe combines various nuts and fruits, adding plenty of flavor and great healthy fats that work to help you slim down that belly. You'll love the flavor of this oatmeal and you'll be surprised to find that it keeps you feeling full until lunch, so you may not even need a midmorning snack anymore.

What You'll Need:

½ cup of sweetened, dried cranberries
1 ¼ cup of rolled, old-fashioned oats
¼ cup of golden raisins
1 Granny Smith apple
1 cup of water
½ cup of walnuts, chopped
2 ½ cups of skim milk, divided

How to Make It:

Begin by washing the apple. Once washed, core the apple and then cut apple into ¼-inch chunks.

In a large saucepan, add 1 ½ cup of milk and the cup of water, bringing it to a boil with high heat. Stir in the oats, adding a pinch of salt if you desire. Heat should be reduced to low, allowing the oats to simmer for 3-4 minutes as the oats soften. Stir regularly.

Add the chopped apple to the oats. Cover the pan, allowing the oatmeal to simmer for about 3-4 more minutes. Oats should be slightly crisp, yet tender. Add raisins and cranberries. Remove the oatmeal from the heat, covering again and allowing it to stand for 1-2 minutes or until completely softened.

Scoop out oatmeal, dividing it up among four medium size bowls. Top each bowl of oatmeal with a ½ teaspoon of brown sugar and two tablespoons of the chopped walnuts. Add ¼ cup of the leftover skim milk to each bowl. Serve immediately. Makes four servings.

Chapter 5: Great Lunch Recipes to Help You Lose Belly Fat

It's important to eat a good lunch, since it will keep you from eating unhealthy snacks between lunch and dinner. Salads are always a great option for lunch and you'll find plenty of great salad recipes that fit in with your belly fat diet. Enjoy many tasty flavors while working to eliminate more belly fat. Try mixing up these recipes so you don't end up eating a salad every day, ensuring you don't get bored of salads.

Easy Turkey Pita with Side Salad Lunch Recipe

When you need a quick and easy lunch, this recipe is the perfect choice. The turkey offers plenty of great lean protein, plus, the veggies are great for helping you get that flat belly you desire. The olive oil in the side salad is a healthy, fat fighting, monounsaturated fat and the unique extras like the hearts of palm make sure you won't be bored with this salad.

What You'll Need:

Pita

1/8 cup of sprouts
¼ cup of baby spinach
4 ounces of turkey
1 whole wheat pita, small
4 small slices of tomato
1 teaspoon of Dijon mustard

Side Salad

½ cup of hearts of palm
1 cup of romaine lettuce, chopped
½ cup of red pepper, chopped
1 teaspoon of olive oil

½ cup of cucumber, chopped

How to Make It:

Cut the whole wheat pita in half. Spread insides of the pita with the mustard. Add slices of turkey to each half of the pita. Top with the sprouts, tomato slices and spinach.

Wash all the vegetables for the salad. Chop the romaine, peppers, cucumbers and cut up the hearts of palm into smaller pieces if needed. Toss all salad ingredients together. Drizzle the salad with the olive oil.

Makes a single serving.

Shrimp, Barley and Baby Green Salad Lunch Recipe

The curry powder and turmeric add a delicious flavor to this recipe, making it a salad that won't make you bored. The shrimp adds plenty of healthy protein to the salad without adding a lot of calories. The wide variety of vegetables makes sure you get plenty of crunch when you eat this salad, while you'll get some healthy fat from the pumpkin seeds added to the mix.

What You'll Need:

1 cup of barley
¼ cup of fresh basil, chopped
1 tablespoons of vegetable oil
3 cups of water
1 pound of shrimp, peeled, deveined and cooked
½ cup of cucumber, peeled and chopped
1 teaspoon of curry powder
1 tablespoons of lime juice, freshly squeezed
1 clove of garlic, minced
¾ cup of pumpkin seeds, toasted
1 ½ cups of tomatoes, diced and seeded
½ teaspoon of turmeric
2 teaspoons of jalapeno chili pepper, seeded and finely chopped

12 cups of baby greens
½ cup of green bell pepper, chopped
¼ teaspoon of salt
¼ cup of lemon juice

How to Make It:

Bring the water, turmeric and curry to a boil in a large saucepan. Once water is boiling, add the barley to the water. Cover the pan, reducing the heat and allowing to simmer. Allow barley to cook for approximately 40-45 minutes, until the barley becomes tender and the water has been absorbed. Remove barley from the heat.

While barley is cooking, whisk the oil, garlic, lime juice, lemon juice, salt and chili pepper together. Add the cucumber, tomatoes, shrimp, barley and bell pepper to the dressing mixture. Toss well to coat evenly.

On six plates, place two cups of the baby greens on each plate. Divide up the shrimp salad, adding salad on top of the bed of greens. Top with the pumpkin seeds and basil. Makes six servings.

Rainbow Veggie, Soba Noodle and Chicken Salad Lunch Recipe

The soba noodles, which can be substituted with whole wheat spaghetti, adds a nice amount of fiber to this salad. You'll get plenty of veggies from the peppers, snow peas and carrots. The avocado offers the monounsaturated fats you need in this meal. The soy sauce, pepper flakes, peanut oil and ginger really add a nice flavor to this salad. The bit of honey keeps the pucker factor under control.

What You'll Need:

2 tablespoons of lime juice, freshly squeezed
2 red bell peppers, seeded and sliced thinly
1 tablespoon of fresh ginger, grated
¼ cup of fresh cilantro, chopped coarsely
8 ounces of dry soba noodles or the same amount of whole wheat spaghetti
¼ teaspoon of red pepper flakes
2 cups of fresh snow peas, julienned
1 ½ cups of avocado, diced
2 tablespoons of honey
2 tablespoons of soy sauce, reduced sodium
2 tablespoons of peanut oil
1 cup of carrots, grated

2 cups of cooked chicken, shredded
2 tablespoons of rice wine vinegar

How to Make It:

Cook the soba noodles or spaghetti noodles according to the directions on the package. Once noodles are done cooking, drain well and then rinse with some cold water to ensure they stop cooking. Set noodles to the side.

Whisk the lime juice, ginger, soy sauce, vinegar, pepper flakes and honey together in a large bowl. Add the peanut oil in a steady stream while whisking the mixture. After dressing is well mixed, fold the bell peppers, avocado, noodles, cilantro, snow peas, carrots and chicken into the dressing. Serve immediately or chill and serve later. Makes six servings.

Mediterranean Style Wraps Lunch Recipe

The olive tapenade that is used in these wraps is an excellent source of monounsaturated fats, boosting the belly busting power of these tasty wraps. The chickpeas offer great protein to the wraps, while you'll get plenty of crunch from the peppers, onions and greens. The lemon juice and goat cheese makes these wraps full of incredible flavor. Make them the night before and take them to work for a healthy lunch that will keep you from eating out and ruining your belly fat diet.

What You'll Need:

4 cups of salad greens of choice
½ of a small red onion, sliced thinly
½ cup of canned chickpeas, no salt added, drained and rinsed
½ cup of green olive tapenade
2 ounces of goat cheese, crumbled
2 tablespoons of lemon juice, freshly squeezed
½ cup of jarred roasted red peppers, drained, sliced and dried
4 whole wheat tortillas or wraps (8-inches)
½ cup of seedless cucumber, sliced thinly

How to Make It:

In a large bowl, mix the lemon juice and green olive tapenade together with a fork. Add the peppers, onion, cucumber, greens and chickpeas to the mix, tossing to ensure they are well mixed. Add the goat cheese to the bowl, tossing gently to avoid breaking up the cheese further.

Warm the tortillas or wraps according to the directions on the package. Place a quarter of the mixture on the bottom of one of the wraps, rolling up securely. Cut the wrap in half at an angle, using a toothpick to keep the wraps together. Do the same thing with each of the wraps. Makes four servings.

Low Sugar Strawberry and Peanut Butter Wraps Lunch Recipe

Peanut butter and jelly is a timeless classic that is a favorite among kids and adults alike. This recipe brings you all the flavor that comes with a peanut butter and jelly sandwich. However, since it uses fruit instead of jelly, you don't have to worry about a meal that includes a lot of unneeded sugar. Also, the wraps add plenty of fiber to the meal, helping you stay full throughout the afternoon. Make these wraps to take to work and make a few extras for the kids as well. Everyone is sure to enjoy these healthy wraps that also help to shrink your belly.

What You'll Need:

1 cup of strawberries, sliced
2 8-inch whole wheat tortillas
4 tablespoons of natural crunchy peanut butter, preferably unsalted

How to Make It:

Place the tortillas on a work area. Spread each tortilla with half of the peanut butter, spreading carefully to avoid tearing the tortilla with the nuts in the peanut butter. Cover each tortilla with half of the strawberry slices. Roll each tortilla up. Slice diagonally into three sections. Makes two servings.

Easy Whole Wheat Muffin Pizzas Lunch Recipe

Whole wheat English muffins are much better for you than white ones, offering more fiber and a low calorie count. If you enjoy pizza, this is a great way to enjoy some of the wonderful flavors of pizza while sticking to your belly fat diet. You'll get delicious cheeses, great flavor from the basil and plenty of belly fat fighting healthy fats from the black tapenade used on the pizzas. They are easy to make and ready in no time, meaning you'll have a nice weekend lunch ready in a flash.

What You'll Need:

1 tomato, cut up into eight slices
4 teaspoons of Parmesan cheese, grated
½ cup of black tapenade
8 basil leaves, fresh
1 cup of reduced fat mozzarella cheese, shredded
4 whole wheat English muffins, split in half

How to Make It:

Preheat oven to 400F.

After splitting the English muffins, toast them. Once toasted, each muffin half should be spread with about a tablespoon of the black tapenade. 1 tomato slice should go on each muffin half. Top the tomatoes with a ½ teaspoon of Parmesan cheese and about 2 tablespoons of the mozzarella.

Place each English muffin half on a baking sheet. Place pizzas in the oven, allowing to take for 6-8 minutes, ensuring that the cheese is well melted. Remove from the oven, topping with a leaf of basil before serving. Serve right away. Makes four servings. You can also make extras and store them in the fridge for a couple days. They make a great snack.

Walnut and Radish Spinach Salad Lunch Recipe

While the walnuts and olive oil add the important monounsaturated fats to this recipe, the baby spinach and radishes offer plenty of important nutrients for the body. The lemon juice, white wine vinegar and black pepper produce plenty of great flavor. Not only does this salad make a wonderful lunch recipe, but it's a nice side dish that can be served up with dinner as well.

What You'll Need:

4 medium sized radishes, sliced thinly
1 tablespoon of lemon juice, freshly squeezed
¼ cup of extra virgin olive oil
½ cup of walnuts, halved
2 teaspoons of white wine vinegar
5 ounces of baby spinach
Black pepper, freshly ground, to taste
Salt, to taste

How to Make It:

Whisk the vinegar and lemon juice together in a large bowl. Add pepper and salt to taste. Slowly pour in the olive oil, whisking continually.

Right before serving, toss the radishes and spinach with the dressing, coating greens completely. Divide up the salad among four different salad plates. Top the salad with walnuts. Serve right away. Makes four servings.

Chapter 6: Flat Belly Diet Dinner Recipes

Eating a good dinner will help you avoid those late night snack cravings, which can quickly sabotage your belly fat diet. All of these recipes include some form of monounsaturated fat, which helps to blast away that belly fat that you are working so hard to lose. You'll find great fish recipes, meatless recipes and more. Even if you need a dinner in a hurry, you'll find easy, fast recipes that allow you to eat a healthy dinner, even on your busiest days.

Smoked Salmon Frittata Dinner Recipe

It's always nice to have a breakfast style recipe for dinner. This dinner recipe makes use of eggs and salmon, ensuring you get plenty of protein. The salmon is full of healthy Omega-3s, which are important if you want to enjoy a flatter belly. The combination of protein and healthy fats help ensure you won't be reaching for a late night snack later in the evening.

What You'll Need:

4 eggs
6 egg whites
2 ounces of smoked salmon, thinly sliced and cut into pieces (about ½-inch wide)
6 scallions, trimmed and chopped coarsely
¼ cup of cold water
¾ cup of black olive tapenade
½ teaspoon of salt
1 ½ teaspoons of fresh tarragon, chopped
2 teaspoons of extra virgin olive oil
Black pepper, freshly ground

How to Make It:

Preheat oven to 350F.

On medium heat, heat up an 8-inch skillet that is ovenproof, heating on medium for about a minute. Place olive oil in the skillet, adding scallions to the oil. Sauté the scallions until they are soft, stirring regularly.

Whisk the tarragon, salt, egg whites, water and eggs together in a medium sized bowl. Add black pepper to taste. Pour the egg mixture into the skillet, topping with the pieces of salmon. Allow to cook for about two minutes, stirring from time to time, allowing eggs to set partially.

Place the skillet with the egg mixture into the oven, allowing to cook for 6-8 minutes. Eggs should be puffed, firm and golden brown on top. Remove the skillet from the oven. Release the frittata from the skillet with a spatula. Slide carefully onto a serving platter that has been warmed.

On six plates, spread about two tablespoons of the black olive tapenade. Top the tapenade with a slice of frittata. Eat immediately while hot. Makes six servings.

Chicken Breast with Almond Crust Dinner Recipe

Chicken packs a powerful protein punch, but it's lower in fat than certain other meats, as long as you don't use the skin. This recipe calls for skinless and boneless chicken breasts, so you don't have to worry about removing the skin. The almond crust makes the chicken something special and also keeps the inside from drying out while you cook it. Serve up with some tomatoes and cottage cheese on the side for a wonderful meal that will keep you feeling satisfied. Keep in mind, this recipe is only for a single serving, so if you're feeling a family or guests, you may need to make extra to fit your needs.

What You'll Need:

1 tablespoon of cornstarch
2 tablespoons of almonds, chopped finely
¼ cup of egg substitute, fat free
5 ounces of skinless, boneless chicken breast

How to Make It:

Sprinkle chicken breasts generously with cornstarch on both sides. After nicely coated with the cornstarch, dip the chicken breast into the egg substitute, ensuring it's well coated. After coated with the egg substitute, sprinkle the chopped almonds over the chicken on both sides.

Spray nonstick cooking spray on a nonstick skillet, heating it up on medium. Place chicken breast in the skilled, cooking for about five minutes per side until done. The thickest part of the chicken breast should reach 165 degrees F to make it safe to consume. Makes a single serving.

Easy Belly Busting Slow Cooker Chili Dinner Recipe

This chili recipe is so easy to make. Since you can put it in the slow cooker, it makes dinner so easy for busy individuals that want a meal that is ready to eat for dinner. With olive oil and avocados, you're getting the fat busting monounsaturated fats that you need. The chili beans add extra protein to the chili and instead of meat, soy crumbles are used, allowing you to enjoy a nice, meat-free dish from time to time.

What You'll Need:

1 can of chili beans (14 oz.), drained and rinsed
1 tablespoon of extra virgin olive oil
1 green bell pepper, seeded and then diced
Chili powder to taste
1 cup of avocado, chopped
1 can of whole tomatoes, salt free (28 oz.)
1 tablespoon of onion, minced
12 ounces of soy crumbles, fat free

How to Make It:

Combine the soy crumbles, onion, oil, chili powder, pepper, tomatoes and beans in a four quart slow cooker.

Cover the slow cooker, cooking on low for 8-10 hours or on high for 4-6 hours. Chili should be well thickened by the time it's done cooking. Scoop chili into four bowls. Top with avocado pieces and serve hot. Makes four servings.

Snow Peas and Steamed Gingered Salmon Dinner Recipe

Salmon is a great protein choice to eat while you are trying to slim down that belly. Not only does it provide a low calorie form of protein, but it also includes healthy fats that help to eliminate that belly fat. The sesame oil, lime juice, ginger, garlic and soy sauce all make a delicious glaze that provides the great flavor for this steamed salmon. Chopped avocado adds even more healthy fats to the meal and the snow peas round it out to be an easy meal that won't take long to fix for dinner.

What You'll Need:

1 clove of garlic, minced
1 cup of avocado, chopped
1 teaspoon of fresh ginger, grated
2 scallions, sliced thinly
1 tablespoon of lime juice, freshly squeezed
1 pound of trimmed snow peas
1 teaspoon of toasted sesame oil
2 teaspoons of soy sauce, reduced sodium
4 salmon fillets, skinless and about 1.5 inches thick

How to Make It:

Rub the garlic and ginger on the salmon fillets. Use nonstick cooking spray to coat a steaming basket. Place the salmon fillets into the basket. Bring about two inches of water to boiling in a large saucepan. Add the steamer basket to the pan, covering and allowing the salmon to steam for about 7-9 minutes.

While the salmon is steaming, whisk the soy sauce, scallions, oil and lime juice together in a small bowl, setting to the side for later.

Once the salmon has been steaming for 7-9 minutes, add the snow peas on top of the salmon in the steamer basket. Allow the peas and salmon to steam for another 4-5 minutes, making sure that salmon is well cooked and the peas are tender yet crispy.

On four plates, arrange snow peas to make a bed for the salmon. Top the snow peas with the salmon. Top each salmon fillet with some of the avocado pieces. Drizzle with the soy sauce mixture. Serve right away while hot. Makes four servings.

Chicken Roulade Stuffed with Spinach Dinner Recipe

Not only does this delicious chicken recipe taste amazing, but it looks great served up on dinner plates as well. It's easy enough to make for a family dinner at home. However, it's elegant enough to make for guests as well. Enjoy plenty of flavor with the red pepper flakes and the sun dried tomatoes. The spinach adds plenty of nutrition to this healthy dish as well.

What You'll Need:

2 teaspoons of olive oil
½ cup of dry white wine or chicken broth
¼ cup of onion, finely chopped
¼ cup of Parmesan cheese, grated
1 10oz package of frozen chopped spinach
1/3 teaspoon of red pepper flakes
2 tablespoons of dry packed sun dried tomatoes, chopped
1 clove of garlic, grated or crushed
4 chicken breast halves, carefully trimmed and pounded into very thin cutlets

How to Make It:

Make the frozen spinach according to the directions on the package. Once cooked, place spinach in a strainer, using a spoon to help press out the extra liquid. You should have about ½ cup of spinach left.

While spinach is cooking, place a teaspoon of the olive oil in a nonstick skillet, heating on medium heat. Add the garlic, onion, 1 tablespoon of water and the red pepper flakes to the skillet. Allow to cook until onion begins to sizzle. Reduce heat to low, covering and allowing to cook until the onion is softened, which should take about 2-4 minutes. Stir once while cooking.

When spinach is ready, stir the spinach, cheese and onion mixture together in a little bowl. Keep the skillet to the side to use later.

On the smooth side of the chicken cutlets, sprinkle with the tomatoes. Divide the spinach mixture, spreading it evenly on each cutlet. Leave about an inch at the narrow end without the spread. Roll up the chicken cutlets loosely, using a wooden toothpick to secure it.

Add the rest of the olive oil to the previously used skilled. Heat oil on medium heat, adding the chicken to the skillet, browning chicken on every side for about 10 minutes. Add the dry white wine to the skillet, covering the skillet and allowing the chicken to cook on low for another 7-8 minutes. Uncover the pan, moving chicken to a warm serving dish. Use foil to cover the chicken, keeping it warm until serving.

Bring the leftover juices in the skillet to a boil until you have a nice glaze. This should take approximately 4-5 minutes. Slice the chicken roulades diagonally into pieces about an inch thick. Drizzle with the glaze and then serve while warm. Makes four servings.

Easy Whole Wheat Veggie Pizza Recipe

As you work hard to lose belly fat, you still do not want to give up some of your favorite foods. The good news is that you can still enjoy having pizza while you are on the flat belly diet. This recipe makes use of many great veggies that will fill you up while allowing you to enjoy some pizza. The mixture of mozzarella cheese, Parmesan cheese, basil, mushrooms, peppers and pesto will provide you with plenty of great flavor as you enjoy this delicious pizza dish.

What You'll Need:

½ cup of finely sliced red onion
¾ cup of cherry tomatoes, quartered
¼ cup of sun-dried tomato pesto
2 tablespoons of Parmesan cheese, grated
2 teaspoons of olive oil
1 cup of button mushrooms, sliced
1 cup of sliced zucchini
½ cup of basil leaves, thinly sliced
1 cup of yellow or orange bell peppers, sliced thinly
1 whole wheat pizza crust, thin

How to Make It:

Begin by preheating the oven to 425F.

Work the whole wheat pizza crust out on the pizza pan, ensuring the entire pan is covered with the crust. Take the pesto and spread it out evenly over the crust. Place the peppers, onion, mushrooms and zucchini in a bowl. Pour in the olive oil. Toss the vegetables in the olive oil until they are coated.

Place veggies in a skillet heated over medium heat. Saute the vegetables for 5-8 minutes or until the veggies have turned soft and the liquid from the veggies has evaporated.

Sprinkle the cheeses over the crust, making sure the crust is covered evenly. Take the sautéed veggies and add them to the pizza crust on top of the cheese. Top the pizza with the tomato pieces.

Place the pizza in the oven, allowing to bake for 18-20 minutes. The crust should be baked throughout and should be crisped slightly on the bottom. Remove from the oven. While hot, sprinkle the pizza with the sliced basil leaves. Allow to stand for 5 minutes. Cut the pizza into quarters and then serve. Makes four servings.

Roasted Pepper and Portobello Mushroom Burgers Recipe

If you find yourself craving the delicious flavor of a burger while you are following the flat belly diet, you will definitely love this tasty recipe. You do not have to worry about the calories and fat that comes with beef, since no meat is used within this recipe. Portobello mushroom caps make up the burger part of the recipes and these mushrooms are full of rich, delicious flavor that will let you enjoy the flavor of a burger without all the fat and calories. The addition of roasted bell peppers and pesto really amp up the flavor, making this a burger that will make your taste buds sing while you enjoy working on a flatter belly.

What You'll Need:

2 roasted red bell pepper halves, jarred
4 leaves of frisee lettuce, or other lettuce you have on hand
4 small to medium Portobello mushroom caps, about 8 ounces
2 tablespoons of pesto, prepared
4 teaspoons of balsamic vinegar
2 whole wheat hamburger buns

How to Make It:

Over medium heat, preheat a large grill pan.

Place the Portobello mushroom caps on the grill pan, grilling them for four minutes on each side. While mushroom caps are cooking, continue to brush with the balsamic vinegar. When mushrooms are nearly done, warm the buns and the bell pepper halves on the grill pan too.

Spread half of the pesto on each of the hamburger buns. On the bottom of each bun, place 1 of the red pepper slices and two mushroom caps. Top with 2 pieces of the lettuce. If desired, add just a little bit more vinegar. Top with the top of the bun. Enjoy immediately. Makes two servings.

Pepper Steak Tacos Dinner Recipe

Eating lean protein and whole grains can help you enjoy flatter abs and this delicious recipe includes some of the best belly slimming ingredients to make a delicious dinner. The flank steak used within the recipe offers a lot of lean protein. You will get plenty of veggies in this dish as well, including bell peppers, corn, avocado, jalapenos and more. Enjoy making this recipe up for a nice dinner. You may even want to make some extras so you can take some to work for a nice, healthy lunch.

What You'll Need:

3 teaspoons of olive oil
½ cup of frozen or fresh corn kernels
¼ cup of Monterey Jack cheese, low fat, grated
2 cloves of garlic, crushed
1 lime, juiced + lime wedges when serving the dish
½ teaspoon of mild chili powder
¼ cup of salsa Verde
3 bell peppers, thinly sliced (1 orange, 1 red and 1 yellow)
1 teaspoon of kosher salt
½ red onion, thinly sliced
½ avocado, sliced
2 tablespoons of pickled jalapenos, sliced

1 pound of flank steak
Light sour cream to taste

How to Make It:

Mix together the lime juice, crushed garlic, chili powder and salt in a sealable plastic bag. Add the flank steak to the bag, shaking up so the marinade coats the steak. Place the marinating steak into the refrigerator for about 20-30 minutes, minimum.

While the steak is marinating, place a cast iron skillet on medium high heat until well heated. Add two teaspoons of the olive oil to the skillet. Place the bell peppers and red onion in the skillet, allowing to cook for about five minutes, tossing and stirring while cooking. Place the corn kernels in the skillet, continuing to cook the vegetables for about 3-4 more minutes or until the peppers become soft and slightly charred. When veggies are done cooking, place them in a medium bowl and place in the microwave to keep warm.

Use a paper towel to wipe out the skillet. Heat the skillet for a minute and then add in the leftover teaspoon of the olive oil. Take steak out of the marinade, using paper towels to pat it dry. Place the steak in the pan and cook over medium high heat for four minutes on each side.

Once the steak is done cooking, remove it from the pan and place on a cutting board. Allow the steak to rest for 5-7 minutes.

Use a sharp knife to slice the flank steak, cutting across the grain. Arrange the steak on a large platter with lime wedges and peppers. Warm tortillas and then begin making tacos. Place steak and peppers in the tortillas, adding avocado, cheese, jalapenos, salsa and the sour cream. Enjoy. Makes four servings.

Belly Flattening Broccoli Rabe Sausage Penne Recipe

Whole wheat pasta is a great addition to your belly fat diet. It fills you up but it does not spike blood sugar like white pasta does. Instead of using traditional, high fat sausages, this recipe uses turkey sausages, which offer a lot of protein without all the fat usually found in sausage. This recipe gets plenty of flavor from the crushed red pepper flakes, ricotta cheese and the Parmesan cheese. The great thing about this recipe is that you can have it ready in under a half hour, making it a quick, easy dinner to use during the week when you are really busy.

What You'll Need:

½ red onion, sliced thinly
12 ounces of whole wheat penne pasta
2 tablespoons of tomato paste
1 clove of garlic, thinly sliced
2 tablespoons of Parmesan, grated
1 medium bunch of broccoli rabe
2 Italian turkey sausages with the casings removed
¼ cup of ricotta cheese, part skim
Pinch of crushed red pepper flakes
1 tablespoon of extra virgin olive oil

How to Make It:

Fill a large pot with water, adding a bit of salt. Bring the water to a boil. Once boiling, add the broccoli rabe to the water, allowing it to cook for about 3-5 minutes. Remove broccoli rabe from the boiling water, placing it in a colander to drain and cool. Once you can handle it, chop it up into bite-size chunks.

Bring the same pot of water back to boiling. Place the whole wheat penne in the boiling water. Cook until it is al dente. Set aside ½ cup of the pasta water and then drain the penne pasta.

While the penne is cooking, place a large skillet over medium heat. Add the olive oil and allow it to heat up. Add the garlic, onion, red pepper flakes and sausages to the hot olive oil. Use a wooden spoon to break up the sausages. Cook the mixture until the sausages are well browned, which will take about eight minutes. Then, place the broccoli rabe into the pan with the sausage mixture, continuing to cook until the rabe becomes tender, about 2-3 more minutes.

Turn the heat under the skillet down to low. Place the drained pasta in the skillet with the sausage mixture.

Toss well to make sure all the ingredients are combined. If the mixture seems a bit dry, add a small amount of the reserved pasta water to the pan. Stir the Parmesan and ricotta cheeses into the pan, removing the pan from the heat and tossing again. Serve the pasta dish right away. Makes six servings.

Chapter 7: Belly Flattening Drink, Snack and Dessert Recipes

Ricotta and Citrus Cannoli Dessert Recipe

Just because you're following a belly fat diet doesn't mean that you have to skip out on a tasty dessert. This dessert will go well with your diet, helping you to achieve the flat belly you really want. Of course, you shouldn't overindulge on these delicious delicacies, but it's fine to enjoy one from time to time. It also makes a wonderful, belly friendly dessert to make if you're having guests for dinner. It goes wonderful with a few slices of banana and strawberries on the side.

What You'll Need:

1 tablespoon of orange zest, freshly grated
½ teaspoon of pure vanilla extract
1/3 cup of powdered sugar
3 cups of chocolate chips, semi-sweet, divided
16-ounces of ricotta cheese, fat free

1 teaspoon of lime zest, freshly grated
2 teaspoons of lemon zest, freshly grated
12 cannoli shells, large

How to Make It:

Combine the vanilla, orange zest, lime zest, lemon zest, powdered sugar and ricotta in a medium sized mixing bowl. Use an electric mixer to whip the mixture together until it becomes fluffy and very light. Fold 2 ½ cups of the chocolate chips into the ricotta mixture, saving the last ½ cup of chocolate chips for later.

Take cannoli shells, dividing up the filling evenly among the shells. Use a spoon to get the filling into the shells or you can pipe it in with a plastic bag that has the tip cut off. Melt the rest of the chocolate chips. Drizzle the chocolate on top of every cannoli. Allow chocolate to harden. Place in the refrigerator. Serve cannoli chilled. Makes 12 servings.

Tasty Strawberry Tropical Fruit Smoothie Recipe

Just a taste of this delicious smoothie is like being in paradise. Enjoy sipping on this drink while imagining you are far away on the beach. Not only does this smoothie taste amazing, but it is good for you. It will help you lose weight and flatten that belly, especially since it adds in some flaxseed oil to the mix. When you are craving something a bit sweet, this will help you fix that craving.

What You'll Need:

1 cup of vanilla yogurt, fat free
1 ½ cup of frozen peach slices
½ cup of mango nectar, chilled
1 cup of fresh strawberries, hulled and cut in half
2 tablespoons of flaxseed oil
1 tablespoon of frozen pineapple juice concentrate, thawed slightly

How to Make It:

In a large blender, place the yogurt, frozen peach slices, mango nectar, strawberries and the pineapple juice concentrate. Blend the ingredients until they become smooth and well combined. Once well blended, add the flaxseed oil to the blender, only blending enough to combine thoroughly.

Pour the blender contents into two large glasses. Add a strawberry half to each glass as a garnish. Enjoy the smoothie right away. Makes two servings.

Delicious Apple Yogurt Dessert Recipe

This wonderful apple yogurt dessert recipe allows you to enjoy something sweet without sabotaging your belly fat diet. You will get to enjoy all the flavors found in apple crisp without the high calories and fat that come with that tasty dessert. The addition of Greek yogurt makes sure you get plenty of protein while you enjoy a sweet treat. Make this for dessert after dinner or enjoy it as a sweet snack at any time of day.

What You'll Need:

2 tablespoons of apple sauce
¾ cup of plain Greek yogurt (or vanilla)
1 teaspoon of honey
Pinch of nutmeg
Pinch of cinnamon
1 Granny smith apple, cored, peeled and diced

How to Make It:

In a small bowl, mix together the apple sauce, honey and Greek yogurt. Stir in the diced apple. Top with a pinch of nutmeg and cinnamon. Mix everything together. Eat right away. Makes a single serving. You may want to double or triple the recipe if you want to serve this dish up to the family as a dessert.

Mocha Protein Health Snack Bites Recipe

If you find yourself craving some chocolate, these delicious mocha bits will help you to quash that craving. Not only will you get your chocolate hit, but you will also get some protein when you eat these bites as well. Keep a couple with you during the day for a tasty, protein rich snack that will keep you going and help you reduce other cravings. They are very easy to make and everyone is sure to enjoy them.

What You'll Need:

6 egg whites
1 teaspoon of coffee
¾ cup of oatmeal
2 granny smith apples, diced
¼ teaspoon of baking powder
1 scoop of chocolate protein shake powder
1 drop of vanilla extract
¼ cup of Quaker oats
2 tablespoons of apple sauce
1 teaspoon of honey
½ teaspoon of cinnamon

How to Make It:

Preheat the oven to 350F.

Place the egg whites, coffee, oatmeal, baking powder, protein shake powder, vanilla, Quaker oats, apple sauce, honey and cinnamon in a blender. Blend the ingredients together until you have a thick mixture. Pour the mixture into a large bowl. Add the diced apples to the mixture, using a spoon to mix the apples into the mix.

Spray an 8x8 inch baking dish with cooking spray. Pour the mixture into the baking dish. Place the baking dish in the oven, baking the mixture for about 25-30 minutes. Remove from the oven and allow to cool.

Once the bites have cooled, cut into eight equal pieces. Makes eight servings. Store bites in a container for up to 3 days.

Delicious Peanut Butter Balls Recipe

Not only do these peanut butter balls make a wonderful dessert or snack, but they pack a great protein punch as well, which can help you meet your flat belly goals. They are really easy to make and once you make up the balls, you'll have a quick snack or dessert that you can grab when you have a craving. Since they have a lot of protein, they will help you stay full and enable you to stick with your belly fat diet.

What You'll Need:

1 teaspoon of vanilla extract
1 cup of Stevia, Splenda or another sugar alternative
4 scoops of vanilla or chocolate protein powder
1 cup of peanut butter, sugar free

How to Make It:

Place the vanilla, sugar alternative, protein powder and peanut butter in a medium bowl. Mix the ingredients together until they are well combined. After the ingredients are well mixed, take tablespoon sized portions and roll them into bowls, placing on wax paper. Once all the balls are rolled, place in the refrigerator until the peanut butter balls are set. Store in an airtight container.

Chapter 8: Your 7 Day Belly Fat Diet Meal Plan

Getting started on a new diet is always difficult, especially when you are trying to figure out how to plan meals so you stick with it. To make it easier for you to stay on your belly fat diet, you can follow this 7-day belly fat diet meal plan. It provides great meals for breakfast, lunch and dinner, as well as some great snack ideas. Follow this plan for the first few days to get you started. Once you are used to the diet, you can mix and match recipes within the book as you continue working to lose that belly fat.

Day 1:

Breakfast: Tomato Pesto Eggs Florentine Breakfast Recipe

Lunch: Easy Whole Wheat Muffin Pizzas Lunch Recipe

Dinner: Chicken Breast with Almond Crust Dinner Recipe

Snack: Mocha Protein Health Snack Bites Recipe

Day 2:

Breakfast: Banana Walnut Breakfast Muffin Recipe

Lunch: Mediterranean Style Wraps Lunch Recipe

Dinner: Snow Peas and Steamed Gingered Salmon Dinner Recipe

Snack: Tasty Strawberry Tropical Fruit Smoothie Recipe

Day 3:

Breakfast: Delicious French Toast with Chocolate Breakfast Recipe

Lunch: Walnut and Radish Spinach Salad Lunch Recipe

Dinner: Smoked Salmon Frittata Dinner Recipe

Snack: Delicious Peanut Butter Balls Recipe

Day 4:

Breakfast: Pumpkin Pie Flavored Oatmeal Breakfast Recipe

Lunch: Low Sugar Strawberry and Peanut Butter Wraps Lunch Recipe

Dinner: Easy Belly Busting Slow Cooker Chili Dinner Recipe

Snack:

Day 5:

Breakfast: Belly Filling Parfait with Granola Breakfast Recipe

Lunch: Easy Turkey Pita with Side Salad Lunch Recipe

Dinner: Chicken Roulade Stuffed with Spinach Dinner Recipe

Snack: Ricotta and Citrus Cannoli Dessert Recipe

Day 6:

Breakfast: Belly Melt Huevos Racheros Breakfast Recipe

Lunch: Rainbow Veggie, Soba Noodle and Chicken Salad Lunch Recipe

Dinner: Roasted Pepper and Portobello Mushroom Burgers Recipe

Snack: Leftover Delicious Peanut Butter Balls

Day 7:

Breakfast: Pecan and Cranberry Scones Breakfast Recipe

Lunch: Shrimp, Barley and Baby Green Salad Lunch Recipe

Dinner: Easy Whole Wheat Veggie Pizza Recipe

Snack: Delicious Apple Yogurt Dessert Recipe

www.ingramcontent.com/pod-product-compliance
Lightning Source LLC
LaVergne TN
LVHW021714060526
838200LV00050B/2659